Year Book of Dermatology – 2019
Trichology

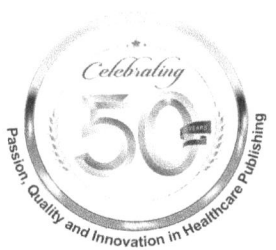

Year Book of Dermatology – 2019
Trichology

Editor-in-Chief
BS Chandrashekar MD DNB
Director and Chief Dermatologist
CUTIS Academy of Cutaneous Sciences
Bengaluru, Karnataka, India

Associate Editor
Madura C MD FRGUHS
Consultant Dermatologist, Dermatosurgeon and
Hair Transplant Surgeon
Department of Dermatosurgery
CUTIS Academy of Cutaneous Sciences
Bengaluru, Karnataka, India

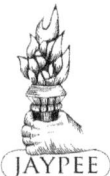

JAYPEE BROTHERS MEDICAL PUBLISHERS
The Health Sciences Publisher
New Delhi | London | Panama

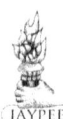 **Jaypee Brothers Medical Publishers (P) Ltd**

Headquarters

Jaypee Brothers Medical Publishers (P) Ltd
4838/24, Ansari Road, Daryaganj
New Delhi 110 002, India
Phone: +91-11-43574357
Fax: +91-11-43574314
Email: jaypee@jaypeebrothers.com

Overseas Offices

J.P. Medical Ltd
83 Victoria Street, London
SW1H 0HW (UK)
Phone: +44 20 3170 8910
Fax: +44 (0)20 3008 6180
Email: info@jpmedpub.com

Jaypee-Highlights Medical Publishers Inc
City of Knowledge, Bld. 235, 2nd Floor, Clayton
Panama City, Panama
Phone: +1 507-301-0496
Fax: +1 507-301-0499
Email: cservice@jphmedical.com

Jaypee Brothers Medical Publishers (P) Ltd
Bhotahity, Kathmandu, Nepal
Phone: +977-9741283608
Email: kathmandu@jaypeebrothers.com

Website: www.jaypeebrothers.com
Website: www.jaypeedigital.com

© 2019, Jaypee Brothers Medical Publishers

The views and opinions expressed in this book are solely those of the original contributor(s)/author(s) and do not necessarily represent those of editor(s) of the book.

All rights reserved. No part of this publication may be reproduced, stored or transmitted in any form or by any means, electronic, mechanical, photocopying, recording or otherwise, without the prior permission in writing of the publishers.

All brand names and product names used in this book are trade names, service marks, trademarks or registered trademarks of their respective owners. The publisher is not associated with any product or vendor mentioned in this book.

Medical knowledge and practice change constantly. This book is designed to provide accurate, authoritative information about the subject matter in question. However, readers are advised to check the most current information available on procedures included and check information from the manufacturer of each product to be administered, to verify the recommended dose, formula, method and duration of administration, adverse effects and contraindications. It is the responsibility of the practitioner to take all appropriate safety precautions. Neither the publisher nor the author(s)/editor(s) assume any liability for any injury and/or damage to persons or property arising from or related to use of material in this book.

This book is sold on the understanding that the publisher is not engaged in providing professional medical services. If such advice or services are required, the services of a competent medical professional should be sought.

Every effort has been made where necessary to contact holders of copyright to obtain permission to reproduce copyright material. If any have been inadvertently overlooked, the publisher will be pleased to make the necessary arrangements at the first opportunity. The **CD/DVD-ROM** (if any) provided in the sealed envelope with this book is complimentary and free of cost. **Not meant for sale.**

Inquiries for bulk sales may be solicited at: jaypee@jaypeebrothers.com

Year Book of Dermatology – 2019 *Trichology* / BS Chandrashekar, Madura C

First Edition: **2019**

ISBN: 978-93-5270-973-1

Printed at

CONTRIBUTORS

Editor-in-Chief

BS Chandrashekar MD DNB
Director and Chief Dermatologist
CUTIS Academy of Cutaneous Sciences
Bengaluru, Karnataka, India

Associate Editor

Madura C MD FRGUHS
Consultant Dermatologist, Dermatosurgeon and
Hair Transplant Surgeon
Department of Dermatosurgery
CUTIS Academy of Cutaneous Sciences
Bengaluru, Karnataka, India

Contributing Authors

Divya Gorur K MD (DVL) FRGUHS (Dermatosurgery)
Senior Resident, Department of Dermatology
Bangalore Medical College and Research Institute
Bengaluru, Karnataka, India

Eswari L MD DVL FRGUHS (Dermatosurgery)
Associate Professor, Department of Dermatology
Bangalore Medical College and Research Institute
Bengaluru, Karnataka, India

Kusuma MR MD FRGUHS (Dermatosurgery)
Junior Consultant Dermatologist
CUTIS Academy of Cutaneous Sciences
Bengaluru, Karnataka, India

Lakshmi DV DVD FRGUHS (Pediatric Dermatology)
Senior Resident, Department of Dermatology
Bangalore Medical College and Research Institute
Bengaluru, Karnataka, India

Nitin Barde MD FRGUHS (Dermatosurgery)
Assistant Professor
Department of Skin and Venereal Diseases
Indira Gandhi Government Medical College
Nagpur, Maharashtra, India

Preethi B Nayak MD DNB
Registrar, Fellowship Student in
Dermatosurgery
CUTIS Academy of Cutaneous Sciences
Bengaluru, Karnataka, India

Savitha AS MD FRGUHS (Dermatosurgery)
Assistant Professor
Department of Dermatology
Sapthagiri Institute of Medical Sciences and
Research Centre
Bengaluru, Karnataka, India

Shilpa K MD (DVL) FRGUHS
Associate Professor
Department of Dermatology
Bangalore Medical College and
Research Institute
Bengaluru, Karnataka, India

Shruthi C MD FRGUHS
Junior Consultant Dermatologist
CUTIS Academy of Cutaneous Sciences
Bengaluru, Karnataka, India

PREFACE

We are pleased to present this edition of trichology in the series of "Year Book of Dermatology – 2019". Trichology is the fastest growing offshoot of dermatology with over 30% of patients requiring services of dermatologists for various hair disorders who attend dermatology outpatient department on a daily basis.

As the subject is ever expanding, a lot of research, clinical trials and innovations are constantly flooding the literature. It's humanly impossible to get the knowledge of all what's happening in the field of trichology. This is an attempt to scan the publications on trichology in the year 2018 and 2019. The book is divided into various sections starting from basic trichology to surgical trichology. The articles are selected on the basis of merit and usefulness to both researchers and practicing clinical dermatologists. We have meticulously scanned over 250 publications and selected most useful 118 articles. The articles are judged and edited by experts in the field of trichology, finally edited by myself and Associate Editor Dr Madura C.

I am thankfully acknowledging Dr Madura C, Dr Shruthi C, Dr Kusuma MR , Dr Preethi B Nayak and Mr Lakshmi Narayana N for their attempts to search the meritorious articles.

I hope and expect this book will meet the expectations of fellow dermatologists, postgraduate and fellowship students of dermatology.

I sincerely thank Jaypee Brothers Medical Publishers (P) Ltd. for their magnificent work in designing and publishing this book. I also thank Dr Reddy's Laboratories for the educational grant for this work.

Happy reading and wishful learning!

BS Chandrashekar

CONTENTS

Section 1: Basic Trichology

1. An Analysis of Gene Expression Data Involving Examination of Signaling Pathways Activation Reveals New Insights into the Mechanism of Action of Minoxidil Topical Foam in Men with Androgenetic Alopecia ... 1

2. Development and Evaluation of Finasteride Loaded Ethosomes for Targeting to the Pilosebaceous Unit ... 3

3. The Effect of Plasma Rich in Growth Factors Combined with Follicular Unit Extraction Surgery for the Treatment of Hair Loss: A Pilot Study ... 6

4. Therapeutic Potential of Stem Cells in Follicle Regeneration ... 8

5. Epithelial-to-Mesenchymal Stem Cell Transition in a Human Organ: Lessons from Lichen Planopilaris ... 10

6. The Unusual Reproductive System of Head and Body Lice (*Pediculus humanus*) ... 11

7. The Genetic Basis of Seborrheic Dermatitis: A Review ... 13

Section 2: Clinical Trichology

8. *Phthirus pubis* Infestation of the Scalp: A Case Report and Review of the Literature ... 16

9. Dissecting Cellulitis of the Scalp: A Rare Dermatological Manifestation of Crohn's Disease ... 17

10. Folliculitis, Tufted Hair ... 19

11. Folliculitis Decalvans and Orofacial Granulomatosis ... 20

12. Head Lice Infestations: A Clinical Update ... 21

13. The Kerion: An Angry Tinea Capitis ... 22

14. Tinea Capitis Mimicking Dissecting Cellulitis in Three Children ... 24

15. Trichotillomania (Hair Pulling Disorder): Clinical Characteristics, Psychosocial Aspects, Treatment Approaches and Ethical Considerations ... 26

16. Assessment and Treatment of Trichotillomania (Hair Pulling Disorder) and Excoriation (Skin Picking) Disorder ... 28

17. Types of Avoidance in Hair Pulling Disorder (Trichotillomania): An Exploratory and Confirmatory Analysis — 29
18. Association between Diet and Seborrheic Dermatitis: A Cross-sectional Study — 31
19. The Correlation between Red Cell Distribution Width, Autoimmunity and Nail Involvement in Alopecia Areata — 32
20. Alopecia Areata: A Multifactorial Autoimmune Condition — 34
21. Renbök Phenomenon: Alopecia Areata Sparing Psoriasis Plaques — 35
22. Linear Alopecia Areata versus Trichotillomania: The Game of Time — 36
23. A New Classification of Early Female Pattern Hair Loss — 37
24. Guidelines for the Diagnosis and Treatment of Male Pattern and Female Pattern Hair Loss, 2017 Version — 39
25. Androgenic Alopecia: The Risk-benefit Ratio of Finasteride — 41
26. Medical Comorbidities in Patients with Lichen Planopilaris, A Retrospective Case-control Study — 43
27. Lichen Planopilaris and Frontal Fibrosing Alopecia as Model Epithelial Stem Cell Diseases — 44
28. Lichen Planopilaris Caused by Wig Attachment: A Case of Koebner Phenomenon in Frontal Fibrosing Alopecia — 45
29. Lichen Planopilaris: Retrospective Study on the Characteristics and Treatment of 291 Patients — 47
30. Premature Graying of Hair: Review with Updates — 49
31. Association of Epidemiological and Biochemical Factors with Premature Graying of Hair: A Case-control Study — 50
32. Association between Premature Hair Greying and Metabolic Risk Factors: A Cross-sectional Study — 53
33. Diffuse Scarring Alopecia in a Female Pattern Hair Loss Distribution — 54
34. Facial Eruptive Vellus Hair Cysts Occurred after 3% Minoxidil Application — 56
35. Alopecia in Association with Malignancy: A Review — 57
36. Incidence and Risk Factors for Alopecia in Survivors of Critical Illness: A Multi-centre Observational Study — 59

Section 3: Therapeutic Trichology (Medical)

37. Controversies in the Treatment of Androgenetic Alopecia: The History of Finasteride — 61
38. Adverse Effects with Finasteride 5 mg/day for Patterned Hair Loss in Premenopausal Women — 63
39. 'Post-Finasteride Syndrome': What to Tell Our Female Patients? — 64
40. Female Pattern Hair Loss: A Pilot Study Investigating Combination Therapy with Low-dose Oral Minoxidil and Spironolactone — 65
41. Clinical Efficacy of Oral Administration of Finasteride at a Dose of 2.5 mg/day in Women with Female Pattern Hair Loss — 66
42. Case Series of Oral Minoxidil for Androgenetic and Traction Alopecia: Tolerability and the Five C's of Oral Therapy — 68
43. An Open-label Randomized Multicenter Study Assessing the Noninferiority of a Caffeine-based Topical Liquid 0.2% versus Minoxidil 5% Solution in Male Androgenetic Alopecia — 70
44. Minoxidil in the Treatment of Androgenetic Alopecia — 71
45. Oleic Acid Nanovesicles of Minoxidil for Enhanced Follicular Delivery — 72
46. Stability of an Extemporaneously Compounded Minoxidil Oral Suspension — 74
47. Efficacy of Topical Combination of 0.25% Finasteride and 3% Minoxidil Versus 3% Minoxidil Solution in Female Pattern Hair Loss: A Randomized, Double-blind, Controlled Study — 76
48. Use of Minoxidil Sulfate versus Minoxidil Base in Androgenetic Alopecia Treatment: Friend or Foe? — 78
49. Off-label Use of Topical Minoxidil in Alopecia: A Review — 79
50. A Comment on the Post-Finasteride Syndrome — 82
51. Low Dose Daily Aspirin Reduces Topical Minoxidil Efficacy in Androgenetic Alopecia Patients — 84
52. A Randomized, Double-blind Controlled Study of the Efficacy and Safety of Topical Solution of 0.25% Finasteride Admixed with 3% Minoxidil versus 3% Minoxidil Solution in the Treatment of Male Androgenetic Alopecia — 86
53. The Post-Finasteride Syndrome: Clinical Manifestation of Drug-induced Epigenetics due to Endocrine Disruption — 87
54. A Randomized Study of Biomimetic Peptides Efficacy and Impact on the Growth Factors Expression in the Hair Follicles of Patients with Telogen Effluvium — 89

55. Study of Vasodilating and Regenerative Effect of the Gel with Nettle Juice intended for Telogen Effluvium Treatment — 91

56. Comparative Evaluation between Two Nutritional Supplements in the Improvement of Telogen Effluvium — 92

57. Efficacy and Safety of a Topical Botanical in Female Androgenetic Alopecia: A Randomized, Single-blinded, Vehicle-controlled Study — 93

58. Tofacitinib for the Treatment of Alopecia Areata in Preadolescent Children — 95

59. Tofacitinib for the Treatment of Lichen Planopilaris: A Case Series — 96

60. Randomized Controlled Trial on a PRP-like Cosmetic, Biomimetic Peptides Based, for the Treatment of Alopecia Areata — 98

61. Tofacitinib (Selective Janus Kinase Inhibitor 1 and 3): A Promising Therapy for the Treatment of Alopecia Areata: A Case Report of Six Patients — 100

62. Efficacy of Diphenylcyclopropenone in Alopecia Areata: A Comparison of Two Treatment Regimens — 101

63. Efficacy of Oral Tofacitinib in the Treatment of Lichen Planopilaris — 103

64. Isotretinoin Treatment for Folliculitis Decalvans: A Retrospective Case-series Study — 104

65. Clinical Studies Evaluating Abametapir Lotion, 0.74%, for the Treatment of Head Louse Infestation — 105

66. Apremilast for Moderate Hidradenitis Suppurativa: Results of a Randomized Controlled Trial — 107

67. Apremilast for Moderate Hidradenitis Suppurativa: No Significant Change in Lesional Skin Inflammatory Biomarkers — 108

68. A Case of Isotretinoin Therapy-refractory Folliculitis Decalvans Treated Successfully with Biosimilar Adalimumab (Exemptia) — 110

69. Turmeric Tonic as a Treatment in Scalp Psoriasis: A Randomized Placebo-control Clinical Trial — 111

70. An Open-label, Observational Study Evaluating Desoximetasone Topical Spray 0.25% in Patients with Scalp Psoriasis — 113

71. Prolonged Skin Retention of Clobetasol Propionate by Bio-based Microemulsions: A Potential Tool for Scalp Psoriasis Treatment — 114

72. Scalp Psoriasis: Report of Efficient Treatment with Secukinumab — 115

73. Efficacy and Safety of 308 nm Excimer Lamp in the Treatment of Scalp Psoriasis: A Retrospective Study — 117

74. Trichotillomania Treated with N-acetylcysteine — 118

75. Treatment of Seborrheic Dermatitis: A Comprehensive Review — 120

Section 4: Therapeutic Trichology (Procedural Intervention)

76. The Effectiveness of Adding Low-level Light Therapy to Minoxidil 5% Solution in the Treatment of Patients with Androgenetic Alopecia — 122

77. Effectiveness of Low-level Laser Therapy in Lichen Planopilaris — 123

78. Low-level Light-minoxidil 5% Combination versus Either Therapeutic Modality Alone in Management of Female Patterned Hair Loss: A Randomized Controlled Study — 124

79. Platelet-rich Plasma for the Treatment of Female Pattern Hair Loss: A Patient Survey — 126

80. The Effect of Autologous Activated Platelet-rich Plasma Injection on Female Pattern Hair Loss: A Randomized Placebo-controlled Study — 127

81. A Comparative Study of Microneedling with Platelet-rich Plasma Plus Topical Minoxidil (5%) and Topical Minoxidil (5%) Alone in Androgenetic Alopecia — 128

82. Comparison of the Efficacy of Homologous and Autologous Platelet-rich Plasma for Treating Androgenic Alopecia — 129

83. A Meta-analysis on Evidence of Platelet-rich Plasma for Androgenetic Alopecia — 131

84. Platelet-rich Plasma on Female Androgenetic Alopecia: Tested on 10 Patients — 132

85. A Randomized Controlled Study of the Effect of Intralesional Injection of Autologous Platelet-rich Plasma Compared with Topical Application of 10% Minoxidil in Male Pattern Baldness — 133

86. Fractional Nonablative Laser-assisted Drug Delivery Leads to Improvement in Male and Female Pattern Hair Loss — 135

87. Microneedling for the Treatment of Hair Loss? — 136

88. Intradermal Injections of a Hair Growth Factor Formulation for Enhancement of Human Hair Regrowth – Safety and Efficacy Evaluation in a First-in-Man Pilot Clinical Study — 138

89. Randomized Trial of Electrodynamic Microneedle Combined with 5% Minoxidil Topical Solution for the Treatment of Chinese Male Androgenetic Alopecia — 141

90. A Pilot Split-scalp Study of Combined Fractional Radiofrequency Microneedling and 5% Topical Minoxidil in Treating Male Pattern Hair Loss — 143

91. Combination of a Nonablative 1,927 nm Thulium Fiber Fractional Laser and Autologous Platelet-rich Plasma in Treatment of Male Androgenetic Alopecia: A Pilot Study — 144

92. Autologous Adipose Derived Stem Cell versus Platelet-rich Plasma Injection in the Treatment of Androgenetic Alopecia: Efficacy, Side Effects and Safety — 146

93. Cellular Therapy with Human Autologous Adipose-derived Adult Cells of Stromal Vascular Fraction for Alopecia Areata — 148

94. Conventional and Novel Stem Cell-based Therapies for Androgenic Alopecia — 150

95. Systemic Photodynamic Therapy in Folliculitis Decalvans — 152

Section 5: Diagnostic and Investigative Trichology

96. Nanotechnology Advances for Hair Loss — 154

97. Parietal Scalp is Another Affected Area in Female Pattern Hair Loss: An Analysis of Hair Density and Hair Diameter — 155

98. "Normal-appearing" Scalp Areas are also Affected in Lichen Planopilaris and Frontal Fibrosing Alopecia: An Observational Histopathologic Study of 40 Patients — 157

99. First Order Derivative Spectrophotometric Method for Determination of Minoxidil and Finasteride in Pharmaceutical Dosage Form — 158

100. Salivary Sex Hormones in Adolescent Females with Trichotillomania — 160

101. Inflammasome Activation Characterizes Lesional Skin of Folliculitis Decalvans — 161

102. Ultraviolet Filters in Hair-care Products: A Possible Link with Frontal Fibrosing Alopecia and Lichen Planopilaris — 163

103. *Staphylococcus aureus* is the Most Common Bacterial Agent of the Skin Flora of Patients with Seborrheic Dermatitis — 164

104. Assessment of Heavy Metal and Trace Element Levels in Patients with Telogen Effluvium — 165

105. Reduced Ferritin, Folate and Vitamin B12 Levels in Female Patients Diagnosed with Telogen Effluvium — 167

106. Color-transition Sign: A Useful Trichoscopic Finding for Differentiating Alopecia Areata Incognita from Telogen Effluvium — 168

107. Trichoscopy in Pediatric Age Group — 169

108. Dermoscopic Findings in Psoriasis and Seborrheic Dermatitis on the Scalp and Correlation with Disease Severity — 171

109.	Utility of Trichoscopy in Tinea Capitis	173
110.	Dermoscopy for Discriminating between Trichophyton and Microsporum Infections in Tinea Capitis	174
111.	A Prospective Study of Tinea Capitis in Children: Making the Diagnosis Easier with a Dermoscope	175
112.	Tinea Capitis in Children: A Report of Four Cases with Trichoscopic Features	176

Section 6: Surgical Trichology

113.	Study of Efficacy and Safety of Noncultured, Extracted Follicular Outer Root Sheath Cell Suspension Transplantation in the Management of Stable Vitiligo	179
114.	Controversies in Hair Transplantation	181
115.	Adipose Tissue Transplant in Recurrent Folliculitis Decalvans	183
116.	Ulcerated Lichen Planopilaris of the Scalp: An Hitherto Unreported Clinical Feature and the Successful Treatment by Surgery	184
117.	Hair Transplantation for the Treatment of Lichen Planopilaris and Frontal Fibrosing Alopecia: A Report of Two Cases	186
118.	Localized Telogen Effluvium Following Hair Transplantation	187

Index *189*

Section 1 Basic Trichology

ARTICLE 1

An Analysis of Gene Expression Data Involving Examination of Signaling Pathways Activation Reveals New Insights into the Mechanism of Action of Minoxidil Topical Foam in Men with Androgenetic Alopecia

Stamatas GN, Wu J, Pappas A, et al. An analysis of gene expression data involving examination of signaling pathways activation reveals new insights into the mechanism of action of minoxidil topical foam in men with androgenetic alopecia.
Cell Cycle. 2017;16(17):1578-84.

Abstract

Androgenetic alopecia (AGA) is the most common form of hair loss. Minoxidil has been approved for the treatment of hair loss; however its mechanism of action is still not fully clarified. In this study, we aimed to elucidate the effects of 5% minoxidil topical foam (MTF) on gene expression and activation of signaling pathways in vertex and frontal scalp of men with AGA. We identified regional variations in gene expression and perturbed signaling pathways using in silico Pathway Activation Network Decomposition Analysis (iPANDA) before and after treatment with minoxidil. Vertex and frontal scalp of patients showed a generally similar response to minoxidil. Both scalp regions showed upregulation of genes that encode keratin-associated proteins and downregulation of integrin-linked kinase (ILK), Akt and mitogen-activated protein kinase (MAPK) signaling pathways after minoxidil treatment. This study results provide new insights into the mechanism of action of minoxidil topical foam in men with AGA.

COMMENT

The pattern of hair loss in androgenetic alopecia (AGA) can be associated with various factors, such as the differences in the levels of hormone receptors and embryologic scalp patterning.

Topical minoxidil and oral finasteride have been approved by the Food and Drug Administration (USA) for the treatment of AGA. Minoxidil is an adenosine triphosphate (ATP) sensitive potassium (K^+) channel agonist as well as a vasodilator. Only one of two forms of K^+-ATP channels found in human hair follicles is sensitive to minoxidil. The drug's effect seems to be connected to its presence and stops when the treatment is discontinued.

Scalp biopsies from the frontal and vertex scalp were done from the leading edge of alopecia and global hair photographs were taken before and after 8 weeks of treatment. Based on a blinded review of stereotactic photographs, patients were categorized as having either full or minimal clinical response. Microarray analysis was done using the Affymetrix GeneChip HG U133 plus 2.0. Pathway activation analysis was performed using in silico Pathway Activation Network Decomposition Analysis (iPANDA).

The analysis revealed that both genes and noncoding RNAs were differentially expressed between vertex and frontal scalp before and after treatment with MTF 5%.

Variations in gene expression in the two scalp regions before treatment were observed. Several genes, including genes induced by oxidative stress and growth factors (*DUSP1* and *CYR61*) and noncoding RNAs, were upregulated in frontal compared to vertex scalp, while the expression of pseudogene *MSL3P1* that may be involved in chromatin remodeling and regulation of transcription was decreased. These results suggest that gene expression in hair follicles in vertex versus frontal scalp of patients with AGA may not be completely identical and exhibit different molecular signatures.

In general, vertex and frontal scalp showed similar molecular response to MTF 5% treatment. The strong upregulation of keratin-associated genes in both the vertex and frontal regions was a distinctive feature of responding patients, while patients who showed minimal response to MTF 5% treatment did not exhibit a similar level of upregulation of keratin-associated genes. The expression of several noncoding RNAs was significantly decreased in both scalp regions after treatment. It should be noted that keratinization-related genes were downregulated in the frontal scalp of both responders and placebo control patients.

Thus, it is not clear whether the decreased expression of late cornified envelope protein 3D (LCE3D) was caused by the MTF 5% treatment or other as yet unidentified factors.

Baseline regional variations between frontal and vertex scalp were also visible upon pathway level examination. Thus, interleukin 2 (IL-2), which is being studied in the context of alopecia areata and integrin-linked kinase (ILK), a key mediator in integrin signal transduction, were upregulated pathways identified in frontal compared to vertex scalp. The following pathways were also upregulated in frontal versus vertex scalp before treatment—Mitogen-activated protein kinase (MAPK) (facilitates the survival of dermal papilla cells), transforming growth factor β (TGF-β) (induces catagen), Janus kinase/signal transducers and activators of transcription (JAK/STAT) (prevents anagen re-entry), phosphatase and tensin homolog (PTEN) and Akt (promotes dermal papilla cells survival and anagen initiation). The downregulated pathways included IL-6), which may provoke inflammation, and Presenilin action in Notch and Wnt signaling (NCI) pathways. It has been shown that activation of Notch signaling is necessary for keratinocyte differentiation, and Wnt signaling drives hair follicle morphogenesis, hair shaft differentiation, hair cycling induction, and maintenance.

The ILK, Akt and MAPK pathways became downregulated in both vertex and frontal scalp of responders after treatment with minoxidil topical foam (MTF) 5%.

The JAK/STAT signaling and Ras pathways were downregulated in vertex scalp of patients who responded to MTF 5% treatment. JAK/STAT inhibition should promote hair growth, while Ras pathway regulates cellular proliferation, differentiation, and senescence by stimulating various parallel effector pathways.

Protein digestion and absorption pathway, which includes several collagen-encoding genes, was significantly upregulated in the frontal scalp of responders. MTF 5% treatment also caused upregulation of mechanistic target of rapamycin (mTOR) pathway in the frontal scalp region. It is known that mTOR pathway promotes hair follicle stem cells proliferation and activation, and is activated at the moment of telogen-to-anagen transition.

> **Key Messages**
> - Vertex and frontal scalp of patients showed a generally similar response to minoxidil
> - Both scalp regions showed upregulation of genes that encode keratin-associated proteins and downregulation of ILK, Akt and MAPK signaling pathways after minoxidil treatment
> - Global response for minoxidil therapy in patterned hair loss is around 42–48%, according to many reports and studies. One of the research could be deficiency or absence or variation in K^+ (ATP) channel pathways and upregulation of gene expressions
> - Also to be noted from this study that minoxidil response is uniform across the scalp
> - Minoxidil upregulates gene expression to proliferate keratinocyte production and migration, and downregulates certain other gene expressions to reduce inflammation.

ARTICLE 2

Development and Evaluation of Finasteride Loaded Ethosomes for Targeting to the Pilosebaceous Unit

Wilson V, Siram K, Rajendran S, et al. Development and evaluation of finasteride loaded ethosomes for targeting to the pilosebaceous unit.
Artif Cells Nanomed Biotechnol. 2018;46(8):1892-901.

Abstract

Androgenetic alopecia, a major cause for baldness, is caused by the deposition of dihydrotestosterone (DHT) at the androgen receptors present in the pilosebaceous unit (PSU). Finasteride (FIN) is a potent 5α-reductase inhibitor capable of preventing the conversion of testosterone to DHT. But, its oral administration in males is reported to have some sexual side effects. An attempt was made to prepare ethosomes of FIN with a size range 100–300 nm to enhance its delivery to the PSU. Finasteride loaded ethosomes (FES) were prepared using an ultra-probe sonicator and characterized for its size, morphology, surface charge and entrapment efficiency. The ability of FES to permeate across rat skin and frontal scalp skin of human cadaver was also evaluated. The spherical shaped ethosomes of different batches were in the size range of 107.8 ± 2.50 nm to 220.4 ± 6.92 nm and showed good permeation across rat skin and frontal scalp skin of human cadaver when compared to the unencapsulated FIN. The results portrayed the ability of FES to permeate across the stratum corneum to reach the PSU of the hair follicle. Although additional use of permeation enhancer increases the permeation of FIN across the skin, its addition may not be a favorable option for the deposition of ethosomes in the PSU.

COMMENT

Finasteride (FIN) is a 5α-reductase inhibitor and targeting it directly is beneficial. Ethosomes are a proven lipid-based nanocarrier to target compounds specifically to the pilosebaceous unit (PSU); the small size, vesicular nature of the ethosomes with ethanol and phospholipids boosts the permeation of the drugs and when used to target FIN at hair follicles, with permeation enhancers like oleic acid, thymol and isopropyl myristate may be beneficial in hair loss. The study attempts to evaluate this action and role of ethosomes. Substrates used are FIN, soya phosphatidylcholine (SPC), Rhodamine Red (RR), oleic acid, thymol, ethanol, isopropyl myristate and propylene glycol. A cold method was used to prepare FES; the average size, zeta potential and polydispersity index of the ethosomes were done using a Malvern Zetasizer (Nano ZS90, Malvern instruments, Malvern, Worcestershire) at 25°C. Finasteride loaded ethosomes (FES) were visualized under scanning electron microscopy (SEM) and atomic force microscopy (AFM), morphology were assessed, later entrapment efficiency was calculated using ultraviolet spectroscopy at 219 nm. In vitro release studies of FIN from FES were done at HiMedia Laboratories, Mumbai, India using dialysis membrane.

The permeation of FES was assessed using freshly excised dorsal skin from a sacrificed male Wistar rat; surface area 2 cm^2 was mounted in the Franz diffusion cell, receptor compartment was filled with 15 mL of pH 7.4 phosphate buffer saline (PBS), maintained at 37 ± 1°C and 1 mL of FES was applied, the amount of FIN present in the receptor chamber was analyzed by ultra-visible spectroscopy at 219 nm. Similarly, permeation of FES across the frontal scalp skin isolated from human cadaver was done using Franz diffusion cell as above, the cumulative percentage of FIN permeated per unit area was plotted as a function of time and the flux values were calculated from the slope and evaluating amount of FIN by spectroscopy. Depth and mechanism by which ethosomes loaded with a fluorescent probe (RR) penetrate the skin were studied in fluorescence microscopy.

Nine formulations were prepared by varying the amounts of SPC and ethanol; additional three formulations were prepared by adding three permeation enhancers. The particle size of FES ranged from 107.8 ± 2.50 nm to 220.4 ± 6.92 nm; when the amount of SPC was constant, an increase in the amount of ethanol from 10% to 30% significantly decreased ($p < 0.05$) the particle size of FES and increased entrapment efficiency. On the contrary, when the amount of ethanol was constant, an increase in the amount of SPC significantly increased ($p < 0.05$) the particle size of FES and reduced the amount of FIN entrapped in the ethosomes. A mild increase in the particle size was seen in all the formulations (FES 10, FES 11 and FES 12) with addition of permeation enhancer. The zeta potential of polyethersulfone (PES) were almost neutral the values ranging from -1.45 ± 0.84 mV to -11.8 ± 2.65 mV. Three dimensional micrographs obtained from SEM showed individual unilamellar vesicles with smooth spherical morphology and the size of the vesicles concordance with the values obtained by DLS readings. Entrapment efficiency ranged $88.4 \pm 3.56\%$ to $62.9 \pm 2.15\%$ affected by amount of ethanol and SPC; highest entrapment efficiency was observed for formulation FES3 containing 30% ethanol and 2% propylene glycol. Addition of permeation enhancer also influenced the amount of FIN entrapped in the ethosomes and entrapment efficiency except thymol. Thus, high entrapment efficiency is obtained by high amount of ethanol, low amount of SPC and a lipophilic permeation enhancer.

The release of FIN followed diffusion and erosion-controlled model with biphasic release pattern ($p < 0.05$) for all the formulations and 25% of FIN was released in the initial phase with sustained pattern of release of FIN from FES for about 8 hours. The cumulative amount of FIN permeated across the rat skin was significantly higher ($p < 0.05$) for FIN when it is encapsulated in ethosomes when compared to its free form (FIN-PBS); Transdermal flux of the formulations were in the range of 67.36 ± 9.23 to 47.92 ± 8.21 µg/cm^2/h, whereas a significantly ($p < 0.05$) lower transdermal flux (39.29 ± 10.3 µg/cm^2/h) was observed for FIN-PBS. In human skin, FES10 containing oleic acid showed highest transdermal flux of 48.66 ± 7.24 mg/cm^2/h followed by 38.47 ± 3.56 mg/cm^2/h and 33.16 ± 5.93 mg/cm^2/h for formulations FES12 and FES11 containing IPM and thymol, respectively. Human scalp skin is comparatively thicker than the rat skin; the amount of FES penetrated over a period of 8 hours across frontal scalp skin of a human cadaver was low when compared to the rat skin.

Fluorescent intensity obtained after application of RES was significantly ($p < 0.05$) higher than the fluorescent intensity observed after application of RR-PBS and RRET. Thus, drugs or molecules encapsulated in ethosomes would show better penetration, however, storage of ethosomes at refrigerated conditions to be considered to maintain stability.

Key Messages

- *Ethosomes of various other drugs meant for topical application would be a good option to enhance permeation to and across the skin*
- *This research paper on ethosomes carrying active drug into the PSU units a novel experiment with high precision and appears to be a milestone in drug penetration enhancer category; ethosomes carry drugs across the skin irrespective of PSU. FIN which is trapped in ethosomes gets diffused in to the circulation which is not a target delivery. The experiments have to be made in developing penetration enhancer and dry trap molecules which enter only PSU, so that systemic side effects of FIN are brought to nil.*

ARTICLE 3

The Effect of Plasma Rich in Growth Factors Combined with Follicular Unit Extraction Surgery for the Treatment of Hair Loss: A Pilot Study

Navarro RM, Pino A, Martinez-Andres A, et al. The effect of plasma rich in growth factors combined with follicular unit extraction surgery for the treatment of hair loss: A pilot study.
J Cosmet Dermatol. 2018;17(5):862-73.

Abstract

Androgenetic alopecia (AGA) is one of the most common dermatological problems encountered in day-to-day practice. Among the various treatment modalities available, only topical minoxidil and oral finasteride are Food and Drug Administration (FDA) approved. Though plasma rich in growth factors (PRGFs) technology has emerged as a promising therapeutic modality in the management of AGA and adjuvant in hair transplantation surgery, there are no well-established evidence for its recommendation. The aim of this study was to evaluate the safety and clinical efficacy of PRGF technology as an adjuvant therapy for follicular unit extraction (FUE) surgery in hair loss affected patients.

COMMENT

Plasma rich in growth factors technology is based on the recovery of a small volume of the patient's own blood which is afterward centrifuged and activated to obtain an autologous formulation enriched in proteins and growth factors. The study involved three in vitro tests and one in vivo study to evaluate the efficacy of PRGF both at cellular level and clinical response. In vitro studies included cell culture and characterization, cell proliferation, and cell migration studies. The prepared PRGF reached 2.29 platelet enrichment over the peripheral blood in in vitro studies and with significant high levels of several key growth factors for hair follicle regeneration like TGFb1, PDGF-AB, EGF, VEGF, IGF, FGFb and HGF.

In cell culture and characterization, the two human follicular phenotypes, germinal matrix cells (GMCs) and dermal papilla cells (DPCs) were cultured in a suitable medium [humidified atmosphere at 37°C with 5% CO_2 with mesenchymal stem cell medium (MSCM)] and the fibroblast-like morphology of cells checked by phase-contrast microscopy showed that both cell types showed spindle-shaped appearance and fibroblast-like elongation. The cells were uniformly positive for standard fibroblast markers collagen type I, fibronectin, and vimentin while showed negative for endothelial P-cytokeratin marker which was confirmed by immunofluorescence microscopy.

Germinal matrix cells and DPC were plated at high density in 96-well optical bottom black culture plates and cultured for 72 hours with culture medium supplemented with 0.2% (v/v) FBS (as a control of nonstimulation) or FBS/MSCGS-free culture medium supplemented with 20% (v/v) PRGF in cell proliferation study. Results showed that PRGF-treated group had high DNA concentration compared to nontreated one ($p < 0.05$). The analysis of migratory activity of follicular cells in response to PRGF showed migration of fibroblasts into the empty gap area between opposite cell frontlines which was statistically significant when compared to controls ($p < 0.05$).

In a clinical study involving 30 hair transplantation, in clinically diagnosed AGA for FUE hair transplant surgery. They were randomized into two groups such that 15 patients received the conventional FUE surgery (control group) while the remaining 15 subjects underwent FUE surgery plus PRGF treatment.

Histomorphometric evaluation (H&E-stained cross-sections) showed the growth factor-rich fibrin preserved pilosebaceous unit along with its associated structures including sebaceous and sweat glands, arrector pili muscle, and bulge region in PRGF-preserved grafts. The immuno-fluorescent images showed that the scaffold provides a natural source of growth factors (PDGF) that adhere to the clot–graft interface and may even penetrate into the FTU before being reimplanted into the receptor area. PRGF-preserved grafts ($p < 0.05$) had high proliferative epidermal cells. The immuno-fluorescence analysis revealed a significantly higher PDGF-weighted fluorescence (WF) detected in the dermis of the PRGF-preserved FTUs ($p < 0.05$) although there were no statistical differences observed between PDGF-WF at the epidermal layer.

Hematoxylin and eosin-stained FTUs showed that there was significant reduction in the structures associated to the follicular unit (such as sebaceous glands, sweat glands, or the arrector pili muscle) and interstitial edema ($p < 0.05$) in PRGF-samples, whereas the 75% of the control samples were found to be seriously impaired. Transected FTUs were analyzed for preservation of the perifollicular collagen. Results showed that PRGF-preserved FTUs presented a higher amount of collagen compared to control grafts ($p < 0.05$). The structural fiber organization in terms of damaged/healthy collagen percentage was also improved after PRGF treatment compared to the one detected in control samples ($p < 0.05$). The orcein stain was used to analyze the elastic fiber. Results showed that the elastic fiber integrity in PRGF-preserved FTUs, 44% of them did not show and 52% showed slight impairment of elastic fiber compared to control sample which was slightly (62%) or seriously (38%) impaired.

Patients were clinically assessed 24 hours and several days after the conventional FUE surgery (control group) or FUE + PRGF treatment (PRGF group). Faster postsurgical crust healing and hair fixation was noticed in PRGF during FUE surgery compared to the control group ($p < 0.05$). The postsurgical inflammation period was also significantly reduced by means of scalp pain, itching and redness decrease in PRGF group ($p < 0.05$). One-year follow-up visits revealed an optimal hair retention status in patients subjected to either FUE or FUE + PRGF intervention. The limitation of study is short follow-up, small sample size, and also needs phototrichogram which would have been more authentic in comparing the control versus cases.

Key Messages
⦿ Plasma rich in growth factors technology is emerging as an important adjuvant in the management of AGA
⦿ It has been shown, in both in vitro and in vivo studies, that the platelet-derived growth factors have significant role in germinal matrix and dermal papilla cell proliferation and also when added to hair transplantation, these provide better collagen and elastin network, early follicle take up, and quick postoperative recovery.

ARTICLE 4

Therapeutic Potential of Stem Cells in Follicle Regeneration

Owczarczyk-Saczonek A, Krajewska-Włodarczyk M, Kruszewska A, et al. Therapeutic potential of stem cells in follicle regeneration.
Stem Cells Int. 2018;2018.

Abstract

Alopecia is caused by a variety of factors which affect the hair cycle and decrease stem cell activity and hair follicle regeneration capability. This process causes lower self-acceptance, which may result in depression and anxiety. However, an early onset of androgenic alopecia is associated with an increased incidence of the metabolic syndrome and an increased risk of the cardiac ischemic disease. The ubiquity of alopecia provides an encouragement to seek new, more effective therapies aimed at hair follicle regeneration and neoregeneration. We know that stem cells can be used to regenerate hair in several therapeutic strategies—reversing the pathological mechanisms which contribute to hair loss, regeneration of complete hair follicles from their parts, and neogenesis of hair follicles from a stem cell culture with isolated cells or tissue engineering. Hair transplant has become a conventional treatment technique in androgenic alopecia (micrograft). Although an autologous transplant is regarded as the gold standard, its usability is limited, because of both a limited amount of material and a reduced viability of cells obtained in this way. The new therapeutic options are adipose-derived stem cells and stem cells from Wharton's jelly. They seem an ideal cell population for use in regenerative medicine because of the absence of immunogenic properties and their ease of obtainment, multipotential character, ease of differentiating into various cell lines, and considerable potential for angiogenesis. In this article, we presented advantages and limitations of using these types of cells in alopecia treatment.

COMMENT

Hair follicular stem cells (HFSCs) form niche for mature stem cells in the hair follicles (HFs). There are variety of factors which affect the hair cycle, leading to decreased stem cell activity and HF regeneration capability, causing alopecia. Dermal papilla cells (DPCs) play an important role in induction and regulation of hair growth and the formation of new HFs. Signals from DPCs activate stem cells in the "bulge" and germinal matrix cells in the late telogen/early anagen phase by activating the Wnt/β-catenin pathway. Alopecia involves changes in both HFSCs and DPCs.

In scarring alopecia, inflammatory cell infiltration around the bulge results in an irreversible loss of HFSCs. Patchy and androgenic alopecia are reversible as the progenitor cells are damaged, but the HFSCs are preserved. CK15+ or CD34+ cells have been identified as "bulge" cells. Stem cells of the upper and lower parts of the bulge in the telogen HF affect the expression of CD34. Cells participating in the formation of a new anagen hair express Lgr5, but not CD34.

Immunoreactivity of CK15 is reduced in patients with patchy alopecia, but is present in androgenic alopecia. There is a decrease in hair follicular CD34 levels in the frontal parts of the scalp, whereas its expression is well preserved in occipital region hair follicles. In patchy alopecia, there is poor expression of CD200 of matrix cells, which is a sign of disappearance of the immune privilege.

The new therapeutic approaches in the treatment of alopecia are stem cells derived from adipose tissue and Wharton's jelly derived stem cells, due to the absence of immunogenic properties and multipotent character, ease of obtainment, and differentiating into various cell lines, and the potential for angiogenesis. This seems as ideal cell population for use in regenerative medicine.

Knowing the mechanism of activation of multipotent stem cells allows their use in regenerative medicine. The effect of microenvironment and expression of receptors on different growth factors complicates its use, and not all stem cell therapy target points have been identified.

Key Messages

- *The new therapeutic approaches in the treatment of alopecia are stem cells derived from adipose tissue and Wharton's jelly derived stem cells*
- *Adipose-derived stem cells seem an ideal cell population for use in regenerative medicine, due to absence of immunogenic properties and multipotent character, ease of obtainment and differentiating into various cell lines, and the potential for angiogenesis*
- *Due to its noninvasive and painless acquisition, ready availability from a large pool of donors, no ethical limitations, no risk to the donor, high multipotential differentiation capability and weak immunogenic potential, Wharton's jelly has become a preferential source of stem cells. Cells can be obtained with an expression of hair-like structures and cytokeratin 19 (CK19) under in vitro conditions. Self-regeneration potential of modified skin is determined by CK19, a marker of bulge stem cells*
- *Tissue homeostasis and damage repair is necessary in maintaining a pool of stem cells.*

ARTICLE 5

Epithelial-to-Mesenchymal Stem Cell Transition in a Human Organ: Lessons from Lichen Planopilaris

Imanishi H, Ansell DM, Chéret J, et al. Epithelial-to-Mesenchymal Stem Cell Transition in a Human Organ: Lessons from Lichen Planopilaris.
J Invest Dermatol. 2018;138(3):511-9.

Abstract

Dissecting cellulitis is a disease of skin with inflammatory origin. The case reported here is of a patient of Crohn's disease with recurrent dissecting cellulitis. A 31-year-old man with purulent scalp lesions presented with abdominal pain, hematochezia, weight loss and night sweats. A diffuse friable mucosa with extensive pseudopolyps was seen on colonoscopy. Scalp biopsy showed epidermoid inclusion cysts with chronic inflammatory cell infiltration and granulation tissue, suggesting of dissecting cellulitis. The occurrence of Crohn's disease with dissecting cellulitis is under reported. Dissecting cellulitis of scalp has a tendency to recur, and considering an underlying condition of this nature is the key for its appropriate management.

COMMENT

Epithelial-to-mesenchymal transition (EMT) is a physiological feature of embryogenesis and wound healing. EMT occurs in pathological processes such as malignant transformation of epithelial cells, metastasis and several fibrotic diseases. It occurs in the bulge of hair follicles (HFs) in inflammatory alopecia like lichen planopilaris (LPP). This study aims at exploring whether human scalp HFs can serve as an instructive model system for studying the EMT process in epithelial stem cells (eSCs) in live human tissue. It also portrays that eSCs in the HF bulge undergo EMT in LPP and that this process may be experimentally induced even in healthy human bulge eSC ex vivo, if exposed to appropriate EMT-promoting stimuli.

In this study, patients with LPP and healthy controls were considered. Lesional skin was obtained from clinically inflamed edges of alopecia; even nonlesional skin was obtained from the patients of LPP. The specimen from the healthy controls was obtained from the occipital scalp. Quantitative real-time polymerase chain reaction (RT-PCR), human hair follicle organ culture, culture of LPP tissue and outer root sheath keratinocyte cells, immunohistochemistry and quantitative immunohistomorphometry and transmission electron microscopy were done.

The authors concluded LPP to be a model disease for pathological EMT in human adult eSCs. EMT signature can be induced and manipulated in human eSCs with peroxisome proliferator-activated receptor-gamma (PPAR-γ) agonists.

> **Key Messages**
> - Lesional LPP HFs display morphological and ultrastructural signs of EMT within their eSC niche
> - Lichen planopilaris bulge epithelium shows an mRNA and protein signature compatible with the occurrence of EMT
> - Cells undergoing EMT within the bulge express the eSC marker Keratin 15+
> - Epithelial-to-mesenchymal transition can be induced in healthy human HF's ex vivo
> - Pioglitazone stimulates PPAR-γ via downregulation of transforming growth factor-beta (TGF-β), protecting against and partially reversing EMT induction
> - The PPAR-γ stimulation by N-acetyl-GED partially reverses EMT signature in normal and LPP HFs.

ARTICLE 6

The Unusual Reproductive System of Head and Body Lice (*Pediculus humanus*)

De la Filia AG, Andrewes S, Clark JM, et al. The unusual reproductive system of head and body lice (*Pediculus humanus*). Med Vet Entomol. 2018;32(2):226-34.

Abstract

Insect reproduction is extremely variable, but the implications of alternative genetic systems are often overlooked in studies on the evolution of insecticide resistance. Both ecotypes of *Pediculus humanus* (Phthiraptera: Pediculidae), the human head and body lice, are human ectoparasites, the control of which is challenged by the recent spread of resistance alleles. The present study conclusively establishes for the first time that both head and body lice reproduce through paternal genome elimination (PGE), an unusual genetic system in which males transmit only their maternally derived chromosomes. Here, we investigate inheritance patterns of parental genomes using a genotyping approach across families of both ecotypes and show that heterozygous males exclusively or preferentially pass on one allele only, whereas females transmit both in a Mendelian fashion. We do however observe occasional transmission of paternal chromosomes through males, representing the first known case of PGE in which whole-genome meiotic drive is incomplete. Finally, we discuss the potential implications of this finding for the evolution of resistance and invite the development of new theoretical models of how this knowledge might contribute to increasing the success of pediculicide-based management schemes.

COMMENT

Pediculus humanus is a blood-sucking ectoparasite, the two ecotypes—*Pediculus humanus capitis* and *Pediculus humanus* differ in their ecology and clinically. The allele transmission in females followed Mendelian expectations, it was non-Mendelian in males: heterozygous male parents systematically passed on one of their two alleles to their offspring. In this study, the authors try to conclusively establish that both head and body lice reproduce through paternal genome elimination (PGE), an unusual genetic system in which males transmit only their maternally derived chromosomes.

In this study, a series of intraspecific crosses was set up using individuals from the head louse strain SF-HL and the body louse strain Frisco-BL. Approximately 50 males and 50 females were used to temporarily establish a colony and approximately 30–50 eggs were introduced each time. Both colonies have been maintained by the Clark Laboratory at the University of Massachusetts Amherst on human blood using the same in vitro rearing system. Offspring (F1) of all crosses were raised until early third instar stage and then transferred to ethanol. Total genomic DNA from parents and body louse F1 individuals was extracted and polymerase chain reaction (PCR) was performed and upon reception of raw trace files, microsatellite alleles were scored using the microsatellite plugin.

This study shows conclusive evidence of a genome-wide male transmission ratio distortion in both ecotypes of *P. humanus*: males exclusively transmit only one of their alleles to their offspring. The heterozygous genotypes in males from both ecotypes unambiguously indicate that males are diploid and that both paternally and maternally inherited chromosomes are kept in the soma. All males in the present study exhibited whole-genome transmission ratio distortion with sporadic, inconsistent leakages of nondriving alleles in some individuals. Allele transmission patterns in louse males reveal that paternal chromosomes are similarly excluded from active spermatocytes, but are occasionally able to escape elimination by migrating with other maternal chromosomes in lieu of their homologues, particularly in body lice. The authors observe occasional transmission of paternal chromosomes through males, representing the first known case of PGE in which whole-genome meiotic drive is incomplete and discuss the potential implications of this finding for the evolution of resistance and invite the development of new theoretical models of how this knowledge might contribute to increase the success of pediculicide-based management schemes.

Paternal genome elimination is present in both *P. humanus* ecotypes and this study outlines some considerations of the impact of the particular genetic system on the evolution of pediculicide resistance. The characterization and compact nature of the *P. humanus* genome enables genome-wide allele-specific expression studies to determine the extent to which paternally inherited alleles can confer resistance phenotypes in male.

Key Messages

- Conclusive evidence of a genome-wide male transmission ratio distortion in both ecotypes of *P. humanus*: males exclusively transmit only one of their alleles to their offspring
- Paternal genome elimination is present in both *P. humanus* ecotypes and this study outlines some considerations of the impact of the particular genetic system on the evolution of pediculicide resistance
- The study may also contribute to the improvement of pediculicide-based management strategies.

ARTICLE 7

The Genetic Basis of Seborrheic Dermatitis: A Review

Karakadze MA, Hirt PA, Wikramanayake TC. The genetic basis of seborrhoeic dermatitis: a review.
J Eur Acad Dermatol Venereol. 2018;32(4):529-36.

Abstract

Seborrheic dermatitis (SD) is a common inflammatory skin disease that presents as itchy, flaking skin in the seborrheic areas. Various environmental and intrinsic factors have been identified as predisposing factors for SD, but its etiology remains poorly understood. Although it was recognized that genetic factors play a role in SD etiology, there have not been studies that systematically review the literature specifically for causal mutations or protein deficiencies in SD. In this review, we searched various databases for gene mutations and protein deficiencies that cause SD or SD-like phenotype in humans and experimental animals, and summarize 11 gene mutations or protein deficiencies that were described in the literature. Most of the encoded proteins play a role either in the immune response [ACT1, complement component 5 (C5), inhibitory κB Kinase c (IKBKG)/nuclear factor KB essential modulator (NEMO), STK4, 2C T-Cell receptor (2C TCR)] or epidermal differentiation [zinc finger 750 (ZNF750), myelin protein zero-like 3 (MPZL3)]. Understanding the genetic basis of SD can impart knowledge of the pathobiology of the disease and help identify novel therapeutic targets.

COMMENT

This review articles summarizes the gene mutations and deficiencies that have been shown to cause seborrheic dermatitis (SD) or SD-like phenotype in humans and experimental animal models.

The authors searched databases—Online Mendelian Inheritance in Man (OMIM), Online Mendelian Inheritance in Animals (OMIA), PubMed, Google and Google Scholar for the articles on gene mutations that cause SD or SD-like phenotype. The authors searched for the terms—SD, dermatitis, seborrhea and sebaceous.

There are handful of studies on gene mutations or protein deficiencies causing SD. To date, only 11 gene mutations or protein deficiencies have been identified that cause directly SD or SD-like phenotype in humans or experimental mouse models.

Out of 11 genes, 4 genes, viz. *ACT1* (*TRAF3IP2*), C5, *IKBKG* and *STK4* (*MST1*), which are identified in humans, are involved in immune functions. The ZNF750, 2C TCR transgene, the rough coat (rc), and myelin protein zero-like 3 (*MPZL3*) knockout and MPZL3 cause SD-like phenotype due to epidermal differentiation changes.

■ MUTATIONS/DEFICIENCIES IN HUMANS

ACT1 (TRAF3IP2)

Two siblings born out of consanguineous marriage developed infantile SD and recurrent oral candidiasis. The mutation was observed in the C-terminus of the SEFIR domain of ACT1. The ACT1 normally binds to interleukin 17 (IL-17) receptors and activates the NF-κB, MAPK and C/EBP pathways upon IL-17 signaling. The mutation causes defects in mucocutaneous immunity by impairing the interaction of ACT1 with IL-17 receptor.

Biotinidase

Two separate cases of biotinidase deficiency with complaints of skin rashes, seizures, SD, alopecia and acidosis were reported. After screening, people who had biotinidase deficiency, daily biotin supplement (10 mg/day) was prescribed, which quickly led to resolution of the cutaneous manifestations and regression of seizure.

Complement Component 5

Complement component 5 deficiency caused SD in two pairs of siblings that presented with Leiner's disease.

Inhibitory κB Kinase c

A 12-week-old male infant since the age of 1 month developed persistent skin eruption with severe intertrigo and recalcitrant SD. He was diagnosed with X-linked anhidrotic ectodermal dysplasia with immunodeficiency. There was mutation in *IKBKG* gene which encodes NEMO, the regulatory subunit of the IκB kinase (IKK) complex that is essential for NF-κB signaling which plays a pivotal role in the regulation of the innate and adaptive immunity, cytokine production and immune development.

STK1 (MST1)

Two Turkish descent siblings born out of consanguineous (first degree cousins) parents had lymphopenia, particularly CD4 T-cell lymphopenia, low serum C4 level and SD. They had a homozygous four-nucleotide deletion (c.58-61delATAG) in exon 2 of STK4. This STK4 is also known as macrophage stimulating 1 (MST1). The STK4 is critical for maintenance of lymphocytes. This is demonstrated in *STK4* null mice which showed severe reduction in the number of T cells due to increased apoptosis.

Zinc Finger 750

Seborrheic dermatitis-like phenotype was found in 44 individuals across five generations in a Jewish Israeli family of Moroccan descent. These affected individuals were found to have a frameshift mutation in ZNF750 (56_57dupCC). The mutation resulted in a putative 44-residue truncated protein of a

C_2H_2 zinc finger transcription factor of 723 residues, rendering it null. The ZNF750 is an important key regulator of keratinocyte terminal differentiation.

■ MUTATIONS DEFICIENCIES IN MICE

Inherited Seborrheic Dermatitis (seb)

The mouse models with spontaneous mutations or induced (transgenic and knockout) mutagenesis showed inherited SD-like skin phenotype. The mutation resulted in seborrhea, rough hair coat, alopecia, growth retardation and rarely abnormal pigmentation in homozygous mutants. On examination, there were neither yeasts nor dermatophytes. These mice model of SD were first animal model which showed a clear mode of inheritance (autosomal recessive), even though underlying mutation remains unidentified.

2C T-cell Receptor

A transgenic mouse model that developed SD-like phenotype had expression of T-cell receptor (TCR) for the cytotoxic T-lymphocyte clone 2C. To study the pathophysiology of SD in patients who are immunosuppressed, this mice model has been beneficial.

Rough Coat

In 1966, the rc mutation emerged spontaneously in a mouse colony at the Jackson Laboratories. These mice had unkempt hair coat, sebaceous hypertrophy, greasy hair, skin inflammation and ulceration which was likely attributed to frequent scratching. This was due to missense mutation in the novel gene *MPZL3* on chromosome 9.

Myelin Protein Zero-like 3

The authors have generated *MPZL3* knockout mice through deletion of exons 2-4. The *MPZL* gene encodes for the conserved immunoglobulin domain. This mutation resulted in the various abnormalities in the skin and other organ systems. The MPZL3 has role in significant function of expression and function in keratinocyte terminal differentiation and barrier function in the skin. It also has role in the regulation of metabolism and energy expenditure, possibly through its localization and function in the mitochondria.

The authors have characterized the persistent inflammatory skin phenotype in the *MPZL3* knockout mice that mimics features of SD at both the clinical and histological levels.

To conclude, author says SD is a common inflammatory skin disease that is chronic and recurrent, with poorly understood etiology. *Malassezia* yeast colonization, sebaceous gland activity and individual susceptibility, all contribute to SD pathogenesis. The authors have studied various genetic defects predisposing to SD.

Key Messages

- *Individual susceptibility, colonization of pityrosporum ovale, and activity of sebaceous glands contribute to pathogenesis of SD*
- *This paper looks into an individual's susceptibility on genetic background*
- *There are 11 gene mutations or protein deficiencies that caused SD or SD-like phenotype in humans or mice*
- *Most of the encoded proteins play a role either in the immune response (ACT1, C5, IKBKG/NEMO, STK4, 2C TCR) or epidermal differentiation (ZNF750, MPZL3)*
- *An extended study of molecular mechanisms on the abovementioned mutations/deficiencies would bring new therapeutic targets for treatments of SD.*

Section 2 Clinical Trichology

ARTICLE 8

Phthirus pubis Infestation of the Scalp: A Case Report and Review of the Literature

Veraldi S, Pontini P, Nazzaro G. Phthirus pubis Infestation of the Scalp: A Case Report and Review of the Literature.
Korean J Parasitol. 2018;56(5):487-9.

Abstract

Phthirus pubis infestation affects buttocks, groin, pubic and perianal region, rarely affects thighs, abdomen, chest, axillae and beard. As scalp involvement is very rare, this case is reported.

COMMENT

Pediculosis pubis (crab louse) is an infectious disease caused by the infestation with the parasite *Phthirus pubis (P. pubis)*. The infection is transmitted by sexual contact, close body contact or, less commonly, by contact with objects. *Phthirus pubis* infests the terminal hair of the pubic and perianal areas. The parasite is not adapted for crawling but can be found in the hair of the legs, forearms, chest or face (including the eyelashes in children). Scalp involvement is unusual for *P. pubis* and only about 20 cases have been reported so far.

Diagnosis is usually based on the typical clinical findings of nits and/or lice attached to hair; severe pruritus, light blue macules ("maculae cerulea") or red papules can be seen at the site of insect bites. The dermoscopic examination clearly exposes the nits/parasites.

This case report is of a 37-year-old Italian woman who had rashes on the nape of neck, upper back following a trip to Vietnam and China. She was previously treated as allergic contact dermatitis with topical corticosteroids unsuccessfully. Dermatological examination revealed nits and lice in addition to excoriated erythematous papules. Microscopical examinations confirmed that the lice were *P. pubis*. The patient was successfully treated with a foam containing 0.165% pyrethrins and 1.65% piperonyl butoxide (1 application/day for 2 days; the treatment was repeated 10 days later).

The reason of the rarity of *P. pubis* infestation on the scalp is unknown. The hypothesis according to which this louse grows only in areas rich in apocrine glands is not convincing, because these glands are very rare on the scalp.

An important difference between the two infestations is pruritus; the latter is very common and severe in *P. pubis* infestation on the scalp.

This case report suggests that although a very small number of patients with

P. pubis infestation on the scalp have been reported in the literature, it is possible that it is misdiagnosed as pediculosis caused by P. humanus capitis. As suggested by some authors, microscopical examination of the lice observed on the scalp is helpful for a correct etiological diagnosis and treatment of the same.

> **Key Messages**
> - Pediculosis pubis is an infectious disease of terminal hair of pubic and perianal areas caused by parasite Phthirus pubis
> - Although it can affect other hair-bearing areas, scalp involvement is uncommon and a dermoscopic examination will help in the correct etiological diagnosis and treatment
> - In an event of uncommon site involvement, one has to study demography of the patient as well as immune status of the patient.

ARTICLE 9

Dissecting Cellulitis of the Scalp: A Rare Dermatological Manifestation of Crohn's Disease

Syed TA, Ul Abideen Asad Z, Salem G, et al. Dissecting Cellulitis of the Scalp: A Rare Dermatological Manifestation of Crohn's Disease.
ACG Case Rep J. 2018;5:e8.

Abstract

The connection between the reported dissecting cellulitis and Crohn's disease can be missed when reviewing mucocutaneous manifestations of inflammatory bowel disease due to the low incidence of dissecting cellulitis itself and the wide array of differential diagnoses. Suspicion of this rare association will help not only in early detection and treatment of both but also minimize scarring alopecia on scalp and strictures and fistulas in the colon.

COMMENT

Dissecting cellulitis, also known as Hoffman disease, is an inflammatory disease of the skin manifesting as perifollicular pustules, keloids, nodules, abscesses and sinuses that evolve into scarring alopecia. It is included in the follicular inclusion triad along with hidradenitis suppurativa and acne conglobate. It has a chronic course with multiple relapses and remissions.

Dissecting cellulitis has been associated with multiple disease entities. It may herald the actual clinical manifestations of an underlying disease process. The well-known associations are arthritis, keratitis, pyoderma gangrenosum, keratitis-ichthyosis-deafness syndrome, pilonidal cysts and osteomyelitis. A rare association with Crohn's disease has been documented.

This case report is of a 31-year-old man with a history of peptic ulcer disease, post partial gastrectomy 10 years prior and antibiotic-resistant purulent scalp lesions for 2 years presented with 5 days of night sweats, weight loss, abdominal pain, diarrhea and hematochezia. On examination, there was bilateral lower abdominal tenderness in addition to multiple erythematous interconnecting plaques on scalp, some boggy with dried yellow crust on the frontal, parietal and occipital areas with scant purulent drainage.

Diagnosis was confirmed by colonoscopy that disclosed severely friable mucosa and extensive polyps along with ulcerated mucosa in the rectum and colon, biopsy showed chronic active colitis and a crypt abscess. Scalp biopsy revealed epidermoid inclusion cysts, ruptured and inflamed, with granulation tissue and chronic inflammatory cell infiltration with no dysplasia or malignancy suggestive of dissecting cellulitis.

The patient was started on steroids and infliximab induction and complete remission of the skin disease and gastrointestinal symptoms was noted.

Considering dissecting cellulitis of scalp, when the patient presented 2 years ago, with a suspicion of its association with Crohn's disease, would have led to early detection and treatment of both, minimizing the risk of scarring alopecia on scalp and strictures and fistulas in the colon.

The connection between the two is often missed when reviewing mucocutaneous manifestations of inflammatory bowel disease due to the low incidence of dissecting cellulitis itself and the wide array of differential diagnoses such as tinea capitis, pseudopelade of Brocq, squamous cell carcinoma, metastatic Crohn's disease and erosive pustular dermatosis of the scalp that can mask the diagnosis.

This case report helps us understand the rare association between the two conditions. Furthermore, the treatment options for dissecting cellulitis and Crohn's disease have significant overlap. Tumor necrosis factor (TNF) inhibitors, adalimumab and infliximab can be used as a bridge to surgery for severe dissecting cellulitis or perianal fistulas in Crohn's disease which result in faster healing and delayed relapse when used after surgery.

Notable point is that, lot of biologics like IL-17, 23 inhibitors can induce or exacerbate Crohn's disease because of unhindered increased activity of TNF-α. In such situation, if one comes across inflammatory scalp disease, the diagnosis of dissecting cellulitis of the scalp should be kept in mind.

Key Messages

- Dissecting cellulitis is a chronic inflammatory disease with recurrences and has been associated with arthritis, keratitis and pyoderma gangrenosum
- A rare association with Crohn's disease has been documented and this connection is often missed
- Treatment with anti-TNF-α can be beneficial for both conditions.

ARTICLE 10

Folliculitis, Tufted Hair

Hughes EC, Badri T. Tufted Hair Folliculitis. In: StatPearls [Internet]. Treasure Island (FL): StatPearls Publishing; 2019. *Last Update: June 4, 2019.*

Abstract

Tufted hair folliculitis (THF) is an uncommon, progressive clinical manifestation associated with scarring (cicatricial) alopecia which affects the scalp. This condition derives its name from the presence of groups of 5–30 hair emerging from a unique, dilated follicular opening. The THF is considered a clinicopathologic feature than a distinct entity rather, since it may be observed in association with several scarring conditions.

COMMENT

Tufted hair folliculitis (THF) is an uncommon scarring alopecia with progressive clinical manifestations. There are 5-30 groups of hair emerging from a unique dilated follicular opening. This occurs as an ultimate stage of follicular injury due to trauma, lichen planus, pemphigus vulgaris, folliculitis decalvans, acne keloidalis nuchae, burns and surgery. It can also occur due to intake of drugs like cyclosporine, trastuzumab and lapatinib.

The THF occurs as fibrosis-induced gathering of adjacent follicular structures and follicular retention of telogen phase hair over multiple cycles. Scarring fibrosis in the upper dermis has been seen on histopathology leading to the convergence of follicular infundibula into single channel; perifollicular neutrophilic inflammatory infiltrate/mixed infiltrates are also seen.

Pain, itching, swelling of the scalp with slow progressive hair loss, with process starting in specific part of the scalp and gradually enlarging. Clusters of anagen hair emerging, as "doll's hair", are seen, with or without purulent exudate. "Starburst pattern" with hair follicles surrounded by white coloration of fibrosis is visualized on dermoscopy. Scalp biopsy helps to assess the underlying disease, extent of scarring and degree of active inflammation.

No satisfactory therapy has been identified, and the treatment is directed toward the underlying disease, decreasing discomfort and to improve appearance. Shampoos, topical steroids, systemic antibiotics (oral rifampicin with clindamycin) and surgical excision of plaques of scarring alopecia have shown varying results.

Key Messages

- *Tufted hair folliculitis has a chronic progressive course with alternating periods of exacerbation and recovery*
- *Not life-threatening, but may have a negative psychological effect due to the cosmetic disfigurement.*

ARTICLE 11

Folliculitis Decalvans and Orofacial Granulomatosis

Męcińska-Jundziłł K, Białecka A, Adamska U, et al. Folliculitis decalvans and orofacial granulomatosis.
Postepy Dermatol Alergol. 2018;35(3):317-9.

Abstract

In folliculitis decalvans (FD) and orofacial granulomatosis (OG), treatment is a challenge as there is no single therapy which can lead to long-term remission. We report a case of a 32-year-old man with concomitant features of FD and OG. Diagnosis and treatment of two coexisting diseases, FD and OG, where etiologies are not fully elucidated till date, need multidirectional diagnostic procedures.

COMMENT

The authors have presented a case report of a 32-year-old man with concomitant features of folliculitis decalvans (FD) and orofacial granulomatosis (OG). The FD lesions over the scalp occurred in childhood and were accompanied by persistent lip swelling for 3 years. Also, skin lesions over the groin, trunk and armpits have been reported. There was increase in C-reactive proteins, erythrocyturia, swabs showed *Staphylococcus aureus* and *Streptococcus agalactiae*, histopathological examination of scalp showed features of FD and of lip showed noncaseating granuloma. Direct and indirect immunofluorescence, patch test, QuantiFERON-TB gold test, antinuclear antibody, lupus anticoagulant, abdominal ultrasound, chest X-ray, cardiolipin antibodies, anti-*Borrelia* species antibodies test and concentration of C1 esterase inhibitor were all negative. The patient showed significant improvement with dapsone, antibiotics and topical steroids.

In FD and OG, treatment is a challenge as there is no single therapy which leads to long-term remission. Regular monitoring of patients with FD is important as there are case reports of squamous cell carcinoma arising within FD. OG may have association with systemic conditions like Crohn's, sarcoidosis and tuberculosis, hence diagnostic evaluation is necessary as done in this case report.

The diagnosis of both FD and OG in which pathogenesis and etiology is unclear needs a multidirectional diagnostic procedure. Fortunately, the treatment of this case with dapsone showed significant improvement.

Key Messages

- Diagnosis and treatment of two coexisting diseases, FD and OG, where etiologies are not fully elucidated till date, need multi-directional diagnostic procedures. No single therapy can be advocated in such situations but dapsone, which is an anti-inflammatory antibacterial, can be a choice of initial therapy
- In FD and OG, treatment is a challenge as there is no single therapy which can lead to long-term remission
- There was significant improvement in these two conditions with oral dapsone, topical steroids and oral antibiotics like gentamicin.

ARTICLE 12

Head Lice Infestations: A Clinical Update

Cummings C, Finlay JC, MacDonald NE. Head lice infestations: A clinical update.
Paediatr Child Health. 2018;23(1):e18-24.

Abstract

Head lice (*Pediculus humanus capitis*) infestations are not a primary health hazard or a vector for disease, but they are a societal problem with substantial costs. Diagnosis of head lice infestation requires the detection of a living louse. Although pyrethrins and permethrin remain first-line treatments in Canada, isopropyl myristate/ST-cyclomethicone solution and dimethicone can be considered as second-line therapies when there is evidence of treatment failure.

COMMENT

Head lice (*Pediculus humanus capitis*), blood-sucking insects that live on the human scalp are a persistent and easily communicable cause of infestations, particularly in school-aged children. This article highlights newer treatment products and reviews more recent information concerning treatment failures.

Infested children usually carry less than 20 mature head lice which live for 3 to 4 weeks if left untreated. The head louse feeds by sucking blood every 3 to 6 hours and inject saliva simultaneously. Adult female louse can produce five or six eggs (nits) per day for 30 days, each "glued" to a hair shaft near the scalp after mating. After 9 to 10 days, eggs hatch into nymphs that molt several times over the next 9 to 15 days to become adult head lice. Antigenic components in the saliva injected as the louse feeds cause itching. Secondary bacterial infection of the excoriated scalp may occur in case of heavy infestation.

Head lice spreads mainly through direct head-to-head (hair-to-hair) contact by crawling rapidly at 23 cm/min under natural conditions. Definitive diagnosis of head lice infestation requires the detection of a living louse. The presence of nits indicates a past infestation that may not be currently active. Without microscopy, the ability to distinguish viable from nonviable nits is difficult, which is why diagnosing an infestation by nit detection alone is not reliable.

Treatment includes topical insecticides (pyrethrins and permethrin 1%), crotamiton lotion (10%) and Malathion lotion (0.5%). Lindane is no longer considered acceptable therapy due to percutaneous absorption leading to the risk of neurotoxicity and bone marrow suppression. If permethrin applications 7 days apart do not eradicate live lice, consider administering a full treatment course using a medication from another class.

New noninsecticidal product containing isopropyl myristate 50% and ST-cyclomethicone 50% works by dissolving the insect's waxy exoskeleton, causing dehydration and death. Silicone oil dimethicone affects the insect's breathing apparatus and is effective against lice, nymphs and egg embryos. Benzyl alcohol lotion 5% is highly effective against live lice but is not ovicidal. Ivermectin, an antihelminthic agent can be given as oral doses of 200 µg/kg spaced 7 to 10 days apart. Ivermectin is not be used in children who weigh less than 15 kg as it is a potentially neurotoxic agent.

A number of household products, such as olive oil, mayonnaise, petroleum jelly, thick hair gel and tub margarine have been suggested as treatments for head lice as thick coating of such agents to the hair and scalp occludes lice spiracles and decreases respiration.

Key Messages

- *Head lice infestations are common in school children but are not associated with poor hygiene or disease spread*
- *It can be asymptomatic for weeks*
- *Diagnosis requires detection of live head lice*
- *Head lice or nits do not survive for longer away from the scalp. Disinfection or environmental cleaning following the detection of a head lice case is not warranted*
- *In case of active infestation, treatment with an approved, properly applied, topical head lice insecticide (two applications 7 to 10 days apart) is recommended*
- *Excluding children with nits or live lice from school or child care has no rational medical basis and is not recommended*
- *Oral ivermectin of 200 µg/kg can also be a choice of treatment but is not recommended below the age of 2 years or <15 kg*
- *Hot combing and blowing hot air dislodges the nits from hair shafts.*

ARTICLE 13

The Kerion: An Angry Tinea Capitis

John AM, Schwartz RA, Janniger CK. The kerion: an angry tinea capitis.
Int J Dermatol. 2018;57(1):3-9.

Abstract

The article reviews comprehensively about "Kerion" subtype of tinea capitis (TC). It is often zoophilic in nature. Oral administration of griseofulvin, terbinafine, itraconazole, or fluconazole along with topical antifungals is the mainstay of treatment. This review highlights new agents evaluated for kerion management and typical TC, enhanced diagnostic criteria, and a grading system for kerion evaluation.

COMMENT

Kerion is an inflammatory type of tinea capitis (TC), mostly associated with infection by zoophilic dermatophytes and often confused with bacterial abscesses due to the purulent drainage. Children, diabetics, anemic, and immunosuppressed individuals, due to leukemia, organ transplant, and the use of immunosuppressants, are at higher risk. Adult women are prone to TC, likely due to periodic hormonal changes, pregnancy, greater exposure to children, menopause and increased visits to the hairdresser.

Clinically presents as a solitary painful, crusty carbuncle-like boggy plaque often at the occipital area. It begins with dermatophytic folliculitis and a dry lesion with scaling and short hairs; erythema, tenderness, and inflammation follows. Localized (Ear sign—erythematous papules and scaling over the helix, antihelix and retroauricular regions) or generalized dermatophytid reactions can occur at the height of the infection. Thus, early diagnosis is essential to prevent bacterial superinfection, folliculitis and permanent alopecia.

Histopathology shows initially neutrophilic and granulomatous infiltrates and fibrotic scar eventually. Four patterns are described, (1) Suppurative type—perifollicular inflammatory infiltrate with spongiosis and infiltrates of neutrophils, lymphocytes, and plasma cells; (2) Suppurative folliculitis with suppurative dermatitis; (3) Suppurative folliculitis with suppurative and granulomatous dermatitis; and (4) Suppurative and granulomatous dermatitis with fibrosing dermatitis.

Authors have proposed major and minor diagnostic criteria and a grading system for kerion. Tenderness to palpation, alopecia surrounding the lesion, numerous pustules and purulent drainage, and scaling at the lesion constitute major features; while dermatophytid reaction, regional lymphadenopathy, short hairs on dermoscopy, boggy plaques, clear demarcation of borders, overlying erythema and pruritus form minor features. If these criteria are present, consult a dermatologist prior to prescribing medications.

- Grade 1: A few pustules overlying erythematous plaque; most hair in catagen phase, but still intact; histology shows suppurative folliculitis
- Grade 2: Pustules and papules overlying erythematous plaque; scaling at the periphery of plaque; few disrupted hair follicles; histology shows suppurative folliculitis with suppurative dermatitis
- Grade 3: Pustules, papules, scaling and erythema present; vesicles may be present; clear patches of alopecia; histology shows suppurative folliculitis with suppurative and granulomatous dermatitis; negative Periodic acid–Schiff (PAS) stain
- Grade 4: Pustules, scaling and erythema present; permanent patches of alopecia with scarring; histology shows suppurative and granulomatous dermatitis with fistulous dermatitis; negative PAS stain.

Grade 1–4 helps in determining treatment response and prognosis rather than choosing treatment option.

However, fungal culture (Sabouraud liquid medium or dermatophyte test medium) is the gold standard to confirm the diagnosis; other culture methods include growth on rice grains, urease test and hair perforation test. Real-time polymerase chain reaction (PCR) test or PCR reverse-line blot assays to detect *T. tonsurans* ribosomal DNA in fluid used to rinse the patient's hairbrush is recent method of diagnosis.

Surgical drainage of kerion is not performed. Antifungals should be promptly started and newer agents, including terbinafine, itraconazole and fluconazole, are equally effective as griseofulvin; should be combined with topical antifungals (1% or 2.5% selenium sulfide, 2% ketoconazole, 1–2% zinc pyrithione and 2.5% povidone iodine shampoos, topical squalamine). Prednisone during the 1st week of infection alleviates pain and swelling, prevents scarring in kerion. Follow-up to be done every 14 days starting with the 4th week of treatment and post-treatment clearance should be confirmed with culture. The recent epidemic of tinea infections show unusual features. Any adult with even mild inflammation should be suspected for TC.

Key Messages

- Kerion is a subset of inflammatory TC that can result in permanent alopecia and scarring. Delineated features suggestive of diagnosis as well as a grading system can be helpful for treatment response also
- The running epidemic of tinea infection requires special attention with respect to clinical diagnosis, drug resistance, dosage schedules, and prevention of recurrence and reinfection.

ARTICLE 14

Tinea Capitis Mimicking Dissecting Cellulitis in Three Children

Shastry J, Ciliberto H, Davis DM. Tinea capitis mimicking dissecting cellulitis in three children. *Pediatr Dermatol. 2017;1-5.*

Abstract

The article highlights a rare inflammatory subtype of tinea capitis (TC) mimicking dissecting cellulitis. A case series of three children, 10–14 years of age, who were presented with an unusual clinical manifestation of TC, that clinically resembled dissecting cellulitis, and were treated with systemic antifungals for 3–4 months. Baseline and repeat fungal cultures, and clinical assessment of hair regrowth at follow-up visits were done. All three patients had resolution of infection, with negative repeat fungal cultures, and complete hair regrowth without scarring.

COMMENT

Case 1: A 10-year-old girl had multiple tender, erythematous cystic plaques and nodules with alopecia affecting nearly 40% of the scalp. A course of antibiotics (doxycycline and cephalexin) was started; incision and drainage done with no success. Fungal culture grew *Trichophyton* species. Prednisone for 5 days and terbinafine for 12 weeks were given, and repeat fungal culture was negative. She had full hair regrowth without scarring.

Case 2: A 14-year-old boy had erythematous, fluctuant cystic nodules and plaques on the right parietal, occipital and frontal scalp with overlying alopecia with biopsy showing deep-dermal mixed inflammation with prominent edema and fibrosis; misdiagnosed as dissecting cellulitis; doxycycline given was unsuccessful. Fungal culture grew *Trichophyton* species. A 14-week course of terbinafine gave negative repeat fungal culture and full hair regrowth without scarring.

Case 3: 11-year-old Caucasian girl with insulin-dependent diabetes mellitus had tender erythematous, boggy nodules and plaques on the scalp with alopecia. She was diagnosed as "psoriasis with superimposed tinea capitis" and treated with clobetasol and itraconazole (biopsy demonstrated hyphal elements). The child was hospitalized and received fluconazole, cefepime, vancomycin and prednisone. Fungal culture grew *Trichophyton tonsurans* susceptible to itraconazole, but resistant to fluconazole, prompting a switch to itraconazole at hospital discharge. Antibiotics were discontinued after bacterial cultures were negative for growth. The patient completed a 4-month course of itraconazole. Hair regrowth began at 2 months and was complete 5 months after treatment initiation. No scarring was noted.

In this subtype of TC, clinically multiple edematous alopecic plaques and nodules across the scalp with minimal scaling in an interwoven pattern are seen simulating dissecting cellulitis, biopsy shows mixed dermal inflammation and inconsistently positive fungal elements, even using special stains. Culture is gold standard, *T. tonsurans* being the most common causal dermatophyte. Authors also enlisted other case series of TC mimicking dissecting cellulitis, which shows *T. tonsurans*, mostly cultured. Treatment with antifungals restores hair regrowth without scarring.

Dissecting cellulitis like TC can be easily missed, misdiagnosed and mismanaged. Increase in awareness of this entity allows earlier diagnosis, prompt treatment, and prevents complications of the infection. Fungal culture is a gold standard and resolves the confusions and burden of misdiagnosis.

Key Messages

- *In changing scenario of fungal epidemic, unusual presentation of tinea infections is rampant. Any scaly patch, postulation or boggy swelling on scalp in pediatric age group should arouse suspicion of TC and investigated as such*
- *In inflammatory alopecia, consider fungal culture, potassium hydroxide examination and bacterial culture in patients*
- *Adjunct treatment with systemic corticosteroids helps in reducing inflammation associated with the infection*
- *Of late trichoscopy should be done in all scalp dermatosis with scaling or inflammations to avoid more invasive and expensive investigations.*

ARTICLE 15

Trichotillomania (Hair Pulling Disorder): Clinical Characteristics, Psychosocial Aspects, Treatment Approaches and Ethical Considerations

França K, Kumar A, Castillo D, et al. Trichotillomania (hair pulling disorder): Clinical characteristics, psychosocial aspects, treatment approaches, and ethical considerations.
Dermatol Ther. 2018:e12622.

Abstract

Trichotillomania (TTM; hair pulling disorder) is a common disorder clinically characterized by recurrent episodes of pulling hair from different parts of the body. Under Diagnostic and Statistical Manual of Mental Disorders (DSM-V), it is classified as "Obsessive-compulsive spectrum and related disorders". TTM is directly related to stress and anxiety. Only few medications including N-acetylcysteine have shown benefit in few cases. Combined liaison clinics, with an interdisciplinary approach, are highly advisable in the treatment of these cases.

COMMENT

Trichotillomania (TTM) is a psychocutaneous disorder characterized by the repetitive act of hair pulling causing hair loss. The disorder was recently changed from Diagnostic and Statistical Manual of Mental Disorders (DSM-IV) (impulse control disorder) to be included in DSM-V and the name "Hair pulling disorder" was added to it.

Actual diagnosed cases range from 0.6%–3.4% and higher prevalence is noted in women. The mean age of onset is between 9 years and 13 years. The scalp is the most commonly described site but multiple sites like eyebrows, eyelashes, face, limbs, pubic area, underarms and chest hair can also be involved.

Trichoscopy shows definitive features in TTM like flame hair, broken hair at different lengths, perifollicular hemorrhage, broomstick hair, etc. When the clinical and trichoscopic diagnosis is challenging, biopsy and histologic examination can be considered. The differential diagnosis includes alopecia areata, tinea capitis, traction alopecia, loose anagen syndrome and secondary syphilis.

Trichotillomania is a highly comorbid disorder, with prevalence of concomitant psychiatric disorder as high as 80%, the common ones being anxiety, major depression, substance abuse, eating disorders, post-traumatic stress disorder (PTSD), personality disorders, OCD and BDD.

Trichotillomania is likely to be the result of the interaction of several factors on a single patient (genetic, psychological, social and neurobiological). A significant association of traumatic childhood events such as emotional neglect, abuse, extreme violence and sexual harassment is observed.

A comprehensive evaluation of individuals with TTM must be conducted by a physician trained in the field of trichopsychodermatology. A detailed past medical history, including personal and familial history, and history of trauma helps in the management.

Some complications that can occur with TTM include repeated stress injury, infections, trichophagia and trichobezoar.

While TTM may be triggered by stress, the habit itself can cause significant stress, low self-esteem, guilt and shamefulness. Studies have shown hair pulling as a disabling disorder, with great impact in school, work and family functioning. Most of TTM patients deny the act of hair pulling and in majority of cases, family members and caretakers also disagree with clinicians. Counseling also to be done for family and they must be told to be nonabusive as well as sympathetic in supporting the sufferers.

Most children outgrow the habit when managed conservatively or with minimal intervention. Adults, however, are more likely to require therapy.

There are no FDA-approved drugs for TTM. Cognitive behavioral therapy (CBT) seems to be the most effective treatment module. Psychotherapy in the form of habit reversal techniques has emerged as an important treatment modality.

Cognitive behavioral therapy appears to be better than tricyclic antidepressants like clomipramine and desipramine. SSRIs and SNRIs have shown poor efficacy in treating TTM. Current evidence shows that there is a scope for using antipsychotics in TTM. Opioid antagonists like naltrexone decrease the urge to pull hair. NAC appears to be a promising therapy.

The concept of brain–gut axis is gaining popularity as it is postulated that the microbiota in the gut communicate with the brain through the vagus nerve by producing neurotransmitters. Probiotics are being used by researchers for OCRD and TTM.

During the treatment process, the physician should have a nonjudgmental, empathic and inviting attitude toward the patient. Recent interest in different pharmacological agents for the treatment of TTM shows hope toward better treatment options. The role of psychiatry–dermatology liaison clinics is extremely important with concomitant patient and parent (in pediatric patients) support services in place.

In mild case, dermatologist should not have hesitance to prescribe SSRIs with low side effects profile like fluoxetine and sertraline. Persistent and recurrent cases should be referred to psychiatrists.

Key Messages

- *Trichotillomania is characterized by constant pulling out of one's own hair leading to hair loss and possibly causing functional impairment*
- *There are no FDA-approved drugs for TTM. CBT seems to be the most effective treatment module*
- *Combined liaison clinics, with an interdisciplinary approach, are advised for the treatment of these cases.*

Article 16

Assessment and Treatment of Trichotillomania (Hair Pulling Disorder) and Excoriation (Skin Picking) Disorder

Jones G, Keuthen N, Greenberg E. Assessment and treatment of trichotillomania (hair pulling disorder) and excoriation (skin picking) disorder.
Clin Dermatol. 2018;36(6):728-36.

Abstract

The article provides recommendations for assessment and treatment of trichotillomania and excoriation disorder (skin picking disorder or SPD). N-acetylcysteine (NAC) is considered for all severity levels and styles because of its moderate gain/low side effect profile. Other pharmacological interventions, including selective serotonin reuptake inhibitors (SSRIs), should be taken into account in cases with comorbidities or previous treatment failure.

COMMENT

Trichotillomania (hair pulling disorder or HPD) and excoriation disorder (skin picking disorder or SPD) are body-focused repetitive behavior (BFRB) disorders categorized by compulsive removal of hair and skin, respectively. It is usually associated with similar conditions like trichophagia, onychophagia and onychotillomania. This study attempts at giving recommendations for assessment and management of these disorders. The current clinical manifestations and the phenomenology of their behavior, any past behavioral or pharmacological treatment need to be assessed. Physical sequelae of the behavior should be managed along with the psychiatric management. Most common comorbidities like obsessive-compulsive disorder, nail-biting or cheek-chewing, body dysmorphic disorders like eating disorders, depression and anxiety should be screened. BFRBs can be automatic, where the person does it without conscious awareness; or focused, where there is conscious involvement, regulating uncomfortable sensations. These are analyzed using assessment scales such as Milwaukee Inventory for Styles of Trichotillomania—Adult (MIST-A) and the Milwaukee Inventory for the Dimensions of Adult Skin Picking (MIDAS) self-report scales. MIST-A-Revised (MIST-A-R) scale includes two new factors "intention" and "emotion". Various other clinician-rated and self-reported tools have been mentioned in this article, which help in assessing change and evaluating progress post-treatment.

The aim of managing BFRBs is complete abstinence. If not possible, harm reduction should be considered. Cognitive behavioral therapy is considered superior to pharmacology treatment. It includes habit reversal training (HRT) coupled with stimulus control augmented with dialectical behavioral therapy (DBT) and/or acceptance and commitment therapy (ACT). HRT does not focus on underlying emotions, and hence they are less effective. It includes awareness training, competing response and social support. Stimulus control training involves limiting behavioral triggers, providing alternative behaviors, increasing barriers for the behavior or increasing awareness around behaviors. ACT and DBT encompass techniques such as mindfulness, emotion regulation and tolerance of uncomfortable inner experiences.

There are no FDA-approved medications for HPD or SPD. Four categories of pharmacologic treatments are NAC, SSRIs, antipsychotics like olanzapine and miscellaneous drugs like clomipramine, topiramate, etc. Clinician should have a nonjudgmental approach. The greatest challenge lies not only in convincing patients of this behavior of them but also in winning over parents and caretakers of patients.

Key Messages

- Trichotillomania (HPD) and excoriation disorder (SPD) are BFRB disorders
- Body-focused repetitive behaviors can be automatic or focused
- The MIST-A, MIDAS, and MIST-A-R are the various assessment scales
- Management involves cognitive behavioral therapy and pharmacology treatment
- Clinicians should avoid compulsive and judgmental therapies and also ensure caregivers' sympathy and empathy attitude rather than commanding, abusive or punishing attitude.

ARTICLE 17

Types of Avoidance in Hair Pulling Disorder (Trichotillomania): An Exploratory and Confirmatory Analysis

Slikboer R, Castle DJ, Nedeljkovic M, et al. Types of avoidance in hair-pulling disorder (trichotillomania): An exploratory and confirmatory analysis.
Psychiatry Res. 2018;261:154-60.

Abstract

The avoidance is an important behavioral feature in hair pulling disorder (HPD) or trichotillomania. Two studies were conducted to identify the types of avoidance and data was collected in internet questionnaires; data from one study was split into exploratory factor and confirmatory factor analysis to analyze different types of avoidance experienced by those reporting symptoms of hair pulling. In the second study, a MANOVA was conducted to know the levels of avoidance that differed between controls and those with hair pulling symptoms. Participants with hair pulling symptoms had greater levels of avoidance on each of the five types: "Avoidance of nonsocial goals", "Self-concealment", "Behavioral social avoidance", "Avoidance of relationship problem solving" and "Avoidance of thinking about the future". These data expand on the current literature, which has predominantly focused on experiential avoidance. Future research will need to validate these findings in a clinical group.

COMMENT

Hair pulling disorder (HPD) is recurrent pulling out of hair in individuals with behavioral disorders and they avoid social, recreational and occupational activities, resulting in a sense of isolation and secretiveness. Systematic avoidance of the behavior referred to as experiential avoidance involves behavioral avoidance, cognitive avoidance, and avoidance in social and nonsocial situations. Individuals with HPD go to extreme lengths to avoid disclosure about hair pulling and avoid intimacy referred to as self-concealment.

In this study, they explored type of avoidance in HPD using Cognitive Behavioral Avoidance Scale (CBAS), The Self Concealment Scale (SCS) and The Action and Avoidance Questionnaire (AAQ). Participants were recruited using online questionnaires on websites popular with cases of trichotillomania. The data set was divided into two subsets for exploratory factor analysis and confirmatory factor analysis. They also compared the levels of avoidance with controls that were recruited by posting links on Australian sites only. The Massachusetts General Hospital Hair Pulling Scale was the measure of HPD severity. Depression Anxiety and Stress Scale (DASS) was used to measure general psychological distress.

Findings of the study were as follows—cognitive and behavioral avoidance of nonsocial goals increased as hair pulling symptom severity increased. A moderate-to-weak correlation was found between the tendency to self-concealment and hair pulling severity. Discovery of pulling hair was feared. Individuals with increased hair pulling severity avoided relationship problems. They also avoided thinking about future.

Behavioral-based therapeutic techniques for HPD have typically focused on reducing the behavior of reaching for a hair with little attention to self-related beliefs or beliefs about how one is perceived in social context. Degree to which types of avoidance overlap with depression and anxiety was not assessed in this study. This study will help to guide the therapeutic protocols.

Key Messages

- Hair pulling disorder has been defined as the recurrent pulling out of hair, with repeated attempts to stop the behavior whilst experiencing clinically significant distress
- Five types of avoidance: "Avoidance of nonsocial goals", "Self-concealment", 'Behavioral social avoidance", "Avoidance of thinking about the future", and "Avoidance of relationship problem solving" were experienced by those who reported hair pulling symptoms
- The context of avoidance should guide future therapeutic protocols.

ARTICLE 18

Association between Diet and Seborrheic Dermatitis: A Cross-sectional Study

Sanders MGH, Pardo LM, Ginger RS, et al. Association between diet and seborrheic dermatitis: A cross-sectional study. J Invest Dermatol. 2019;139(1):108-14.

Abstract

Seborrheic dermatitis causes erythema, scaling, and pruritus of the affected area. The current available therapies aim to reduce the symptoms, but the risk of recurrence is always there. Identifying a disease modifiable factor may help in reducing the disease burden. This study was conducted with the objective to determine whether specific dietary patterns or total antioxidant capacity are associated with seborrheic dermatitis. The authors concluded that a high fruit intake was associated with less seborrheic dermatitis, whereas high adherence to a "Western" dietary pattern in females was associated with more seborrheic dermatitis.

COMMENT

Seborrheic dermatitis is a chronic relapsing scalp disorder, where *Malassezia* yeast plays a significant role. Diet plays a role in many dermatitis. Lot of articles are published on relation of diet in acne, psoriasis and hair loss. In this study, authors have found that participants with a dietary pattern characterized by high fruit intake had lower odds of having seborrheic dermatitis. Fruits are a rich source of vitamin, flavonoids and antioxidants. These compounds have been shown to have anti-inflammatory properties. Also, citrus fruits are rich in psoralen and their consumption might have increased the sensitivity to UVR which could have had a positive effect on seborrheic dermatitis. It was also observed that Western diet increased the odds of seborrheic dermatitis in women but not in men. As seborrheic dermatitis is a chronic inflammatory condition, and because reactive oxygen species may promote chronic inflammation, authors speculated individuals with high total antioxidant intake to have a lower prevalence of skin disease. Contrary to that, participants with a higher overall dietary antioxidant capacity did not have a decreased odds of having seborrheic dermatitis.

Key Messages

- *A high intake of fruit was associated with lower odds of seborrheic dermatitis, and a high adherence to the Western dietary pattern seems to be associated with a higher risk of seborrheic dermatitis in females*
- *Dietary modifications in patients with seborrheic dermatitis is a thoughtful way to reduce the intensity and recurrence of seborrheic dermatitis*
- *The observation in this study also opens up possibility of therapeutic intervention of seborrheic dermatitis with oral antioxidants, but requires case-control studies to prove the hypothesis.*

ARTICLE 19

The Correlation between Red Cell Distribution Width, Autoimmunity and Nail Involvement in Alopecia Areata

Gürel G. The correlation between red cell distribution width, autoimmunity and nail involvement in alopecia areata. *Eur Res J. 2018;1-6.*

Abstract

Objectives: Alopecia areata (AA) is a widespread autoimmune disease that targets hair follicles, and is characterized by nonscarring patches of hair loss. Red cell distribution width (RDW) is a routinely analyzed parameter during complete blood count, and indicates variations in diameters of red blood cells. Elevated RDW levels are associated with high level of inflammation and oxidative stress. In this study, we aimed to demonstrate the correlation between RDW levels, autoimmunity, and nail involvement in alopecia areata.

Methods: Medical records of 170 patients who were admitted to our dermatology clinic between May 2016 and May 2017 were retrospectively evaluated. A total of 170 patients with alopecia areata diagnosis were evaluated.

Results: The mean age of the patients was 24.61 ± 12.62 years (3–59 years). Sixty patients (35.3%) were female, and 110 patients (64.7%) were male. Twenty seven patients (15.9%) had nail involvement, and 24 patients (14.1%) had a history of an autoimmune disease. RDW levels were significantly higher in patients with nail involvement and history of an autoimmune disease.

Conclusion: RDW can be used as a simple, cheap, and readily available marker of inflammation in patients with AA.

COMMENT

Alopecia areata (AA) is an autoimmune disease resulting from T cell-mediated damage to hair follicles. The exact etiopathogenetic factors in AA are still inconclusive, yet the role of immune breakdown at the follicular level is accepted beyond doubt. Hence, the biomarkers of inflammation play a pivotal role in understanding the course of AA. Inflammatory cytokines have an impact on half-life of red blood cells and lead to elevated red cell distribution width (RDW).

Red cell distribution width and mean platelet volume (MPV) are parameters in complete blood count which are routinely evaluated; they are also considered as markers of inflammation and oxidative stress. They have been used to predict prognosis in autoimmune disorders like inflammatory bowel diseases, psoriasis and rheumatoid arthritis. This data has been extrapolated by the author to explore RDW levels in AA and also an attempt to correlate with clinical parameters and associated disorders of AA is made promptly.

The article is a retrospective, descriptive analysis of 170 patients diagnosed with AA.

The mean age of the patients was 24.61 ± 12.62 years (3–59 years). Females constituted 60 patients (35.3%) and males 110 patients (64.7%) with scalp involvement being the most common site identified in 112 patients (65.9%), followed by beard involvement [32 patients (18.8%)], eyebrow involvement [4 patients (2.4%)], mixed involvement [16 patients (9.4%)] and universal involvement [6 patients (3.5%)].

Nail involvement was found in 27 patients (15.9%) with mean age of patients with nail involvement was 18.11 ± 11.51 years ($p < 0.01$) and without nail involvement was 25.84 ± 12.48 years. A statistically significant mean RDW level was found in patients without nail involvement and with nail involvement (12.77 ± 0.79 and 13.24 ± 1.13, respectively; $p = 0.041$). The mean ST4 value was also significant, 1.00 ± 0.09 in patients of AA without nail involvement, and 1.11 ± 0.18 in patients of AA with nail involvement ($p < 0.01$).

Twenty-four patients (14.1%) had a history of an autoimmune disease with mean age of 24.34 ± 12.29 years. On analyzing the correlation between having history of an autoimmune disease and RDW, a significant difference in the mean RDW level was found among patients without an autoimmune disease and patients with an autoimmune disease (12.75 ± 0.75 vs. 13.37 ± 1.25; $p = 0.021$). The mean ST4 level was 1.00 ± 0.09 in patients without an autoimmune disease, and 1.10 ± 0.19 in patients with an autoimmune disease ($p < 0.01$).

The mean anti-TG level and anti-TPO value were also found to be significant in AA with autoimmunity. Mean anti-TG level was 107.69 ± 259.52 and mean anti-TPO value was 215.40 ± 383.98, respectively in autoimmune disease positive patients ($p < 0.01$) in comparison to patients without an autoimmune disease (mean anti-TPO value was 15.22 ± 88.19 and anti-TG level was 8.78 ± 64.58).

Hemoglobin level, neutrophil count, leukocyte count, MPV, glucose, vitamin B12, TSH and serum T3 levels were also simultaneously assessed but no significant correlation could be established by the study.

Poor prognostic factors in AA include early disease onset, prolonged duration, severe forms, viz. alopecia totalis and alopecia universalis, nail involvement, family history, comorbid states like atopic dermatitis, and autoimmune disease. Since high RDW has been associated with poor prognosis and severe inflammation in relation to autoimmune disease and nail involvement in AA. Hence RDW adds valuable information and can be used as biomarker tool in AA. As well, periodic estimation of RDW may also indicate activity of the disease, response to treatment and recurrence.

Key Messages

- Red cell distribution width is a simple hematological parameter which can be used as a marker of inflammation in AA
- Better designed studies and control studies are further needed to establish the definite role of RDW as a serum marker.

ARTICLE 20

Alopecia Areata: A Multifactorial Autoimmune Condition

Simakou T, Butcher JP, Reid S, et al. Alopecia areata: A multifactorial autoimmune condition. *J Autoimmun.* 2019;98:74-85.

Abstract

Though alopecia areata (AA) is an autoimmune disease, etiology and pathophysiology of disease are not well-defined. The reason for hair loss is due to lymphocytic infiltrations around the hair follicles. This review discusses various genetic and environmental factors causing autoimmunity. It also describes the immune mechanisms that lead to hair loss in patients.

COMMENT

Alopecia areata (AA) is an autoimmune disease characterized by patchy or diffuse hair loss due to inflammatory response targeting the hair follicles. The exact cause of AA is poorly understood but the genetics and immunity are the most important contributing factors. Pathology includes infiltration of T helper (Th) cells, cytolytic T cells, natural killer cells and plasmacytoid dendritic cells (PDCs) around the lower part of the hair bulb leading to the breach in the hair follicle immune privilege leading to alopecia. CD8+ cells are the main cell type that initiates AA with unpredictable response. These infiltrates disturb hair follicle functioning with premature hair loss and inhibition of hair growth. In this condition, hair follicle is not destroyed, so the outcome is hair fall without scarring or permanent loss of tissue.

Alopecia areata is a heritable, complex and polygenic condition associated with a variety of other autoimmune diseases. The major genes associated with AA are *NOTCH4*, *KLRK1* and *AIRE*. The major immune cells involved in AA are CD4+ T cells, CD8+ NKG2D+ T cells and NK cells. CD8+ NKG2D+ T cells (cytotoxic T cells) have been major contributors and are the first to infiltrate around the hair follicles. CD8+ T cells attack the hair follicle using Granzyme B (GZMB). AA is associated with imbalance between Th17 and Treg cells, with Th17 levels in blood exceeding the Treg levels during active stages of disease. PDCs are a link between the innate and adaptive immunity which is absent in normal skin but can infiltrate upon injury or pathology. Upon activation they produce large quantities of type I interferons (IFN-α/β), which have been implicated in AA for inducing CD4+, CD8+ and NK responses toward the hair follicles leading to release of IFN-γ. IFN-γ causes collapse of the hair follicle immune privilege by expression of MHC-I molecules and ligands that stimulate NK-cell receptors (NKG2D) in the anagen hair bulb. IFN-γ also induces JAK/STAT signaling leading to premature termination of the anagen phase in AA.

Other than genetic and immune system, the other triggering factors for AA include oxidative stress, psychological stress, infectious agents, microbiota and diet. Treatments for AA are mainly focused at targeting this autoimmunity.

> **Key Message**
>
> - Alopecia areata is an autoimmune disease with genetic and environmental etiology. Prevention of autoimmune alopecia is challenging because of the multifactorial etiology, which may require difficult genetic testing and strict avoidance of environmental factors. Better diagnosis of comorbidities and identification of initiating factors can lead to patient-specific therapies that can be more effective than the current ones.

ARTICLE 21

Renbök Phenomenon: Alopecia Areata Sparing Psoriasis Plaques

Gupta M, Mahajan VK. Renbök phenomenon: Alopecia areata sparing psoriasis plaques. *Our Dermatol Online.* 2018;9(3):333-4.

Abstract

Renbök phenomenon, a reverse of "Koebner" phenomenon, is a recent term coined by Happle et al. It designates the withdrawal of a lesion with the appearance of another one. This article reports a 45-year-old patient, who suddenly developed alopecia areata (AA) with pre-existing plaque psoriasis involving scalp and extensor, and experienced regression of a psoriatic plaque on the scalp concurrently with the appearance of a patch of AA. The hair loss in patches of AA was total and spared psoriatic plaques reflecting Renbök phenomenon.

COMMENT

Alopecia areata (AA) is an autoimmune T cell-mediated disease, although its exact mechanism is still obscure. AA is usually associated with other autoimmune disorders such as vitiligo and psoriasis. The remission of AA in psoriatic plaques is called Renbök phenomenon. This article reports a case of 45-year-old man presented with sudden onset asymptomatic patchy loss of hair with plaque psoriasis involving scalp. The psoriasis plaques were well-delineated and stopped short of AA patches without any encroachment and showed normal hair growth. Hair loss in patches of AA was total and spared psoriatic plaques reflecting Renbök phenomenon.

The exact pathomechanism is unknown and it is hypothesized that in psoriasis (Th17 mediated dermatoses) and AA (Th1 mediated disorder), T-cell subsets, by cytokine production, enhance their own response through positive feedback while antagonizing the other responses in the affected areas. Criado et al. proposed that the microenvironment of high levels of TNF-α in psoriasis is not favorable for the development of inflammatory response in AA-producing characteristic Renbök phenomenon.

> **Key Message**
>
> - This article highlights a phenomenon, which is unique in that there is a rapid change from one disorder to the other. The Renbök phenomenon designates the withdrawal of a lesion when a different one appears. Its application expanded to include AA similarly sparing nevus flammeus or congenital nevus.

ARTICLE 22

Linear Alopecia Areata versus Trichotillomania: The Game of Time

Mukherjee SS, Chandrashekar BS. Linear alopecia areata versus trichotillomania: The game of time.
Indian J Paediatr Dermatol. 2018;19:136-8.

Abstract

This article reports a rare case of linear alopecia areata (AA) simulating trichotillomania. Unusual presentation of either of the one will have diagnostic challenge for treatment. AA has varied presentation. The dermoscopic evaluation and careful clinical history and follow-up clinches the diagnosis.

COMMENT

Alopecia areata (AA) and trichotillomania are both common disorders of childhood. Unusual presentation of either of the one will have diagnostic challenge for treatment. AA is the most common form of nonscarring alopecias occurring in children. It has varied presentation ranging from a single patch, multifocal, sisaphio pattern, ophiasis pattern, reticular, diffuse, totalis and universalis, perinevoid, and very rarely linear pattern. This article reports a case of linear AA mimicking trichotillomania.

In this case report, a 7-year-old girl child presented with complaints of asymptomatic, patchy hair loss over the scalp of 3 weeks duration. Hair loss was initially noted over the left temporal area, which further spread to involve the right temporal and vertex area.

Examination of the scalp revealed three linear patches of hair loss with smooth underlying skin; hair of varying length were noted. The dermoscopic evaluation revealed broken hair, black dots, flame hair and V-hair on the patches. Provisional diagnosis of trichotillomania was made and on treatment, the child still had extension of patch which clinched the diagnosis of linear AA. The child was managed with topical minoxidil 2% application with mometasone ointment which showed good response.

Key Message

- In this article, the case of linear AA was missed in the beginning due to the evidence such as excoriations, hair of varying length on the patch, sudden onset and dermoscopic findings of broken hair, perifollicular hemorrhage, and black dots masquerading the picture and supporting the diagnosis of trichotillomania. AA was diagnosed during the follow-up, which highlights the importance of periodic follow-up, an open mind, and a thorough clinical examination.

ARTICLE 23

A New Classification of Early Female Pattern Hair Loss

Kaneko A, Kaneko T. A new classification of early female pattern hair loss.
Int J Trichol. 2018;10(2):61-7.

Abstract

The authors have made an attempt to propose a classification system that helps in grading as well as evaluating the treatment course of early female pattern hair loss (FPHL) based on changes in hair surface reflection patterns. Retrospective chart review of 114 early FPHL patients was performed with global photographs (GPs) and was classified into five grades pairing lowest and the highest grades of each patient. FPHL-severity index (FPHL-SI) and grades of all the selected photos were analyzed by three volunteers and authors. The value of FPHL-SI and incidence rate of hair diameter diversity tended to rise along with increasing of GP grade with a concordance rate of grading among authors being 57% and, that of course evaluation among authors was 97%. Thus, classification is promising in grading and follow-up of early FPHL.

COMMENT

A retrospective chart review of 114 early female pattern hair loss (FPHL) patients was performed with global photographs (GPs) and a grading system for early FPHL with five levels focusing on the changes revealed by the surface reflected flashlight of GPs was performed. Surface reflected light is light which hits the hair and reflects on the surface of the cuticle and appears as shining white; quality of band can be used as an index in FPHL. The authors have used this as a tool in grading early FPHL. GPs with the highest grade (severe) and lowest grade (mild) for each patient (n = 228) were selected and evaluated with existing photographs along with dermoscopy and the FPHL-severity index [FPHL-SI (includes the amount of hair shedding, midline hair density, hair diameter variation, and difference in the proportion of single hair per hair follicle unit between the frontal and occipital scalp)] using data of the closest date to the photographs. Five groups by GP grades were done, and the average value of FPHL-SI of each group was calculated. Two photos selected from each patient were randomly allocated to either side of one slide and evaluated by three volunteers. Then, concordance rate among the author's and volunteers' evaluations was analyzed.

The mean age was 39.1 years (range, 20-55 years), and the mean age of onset was 36.0 years old (15-53 years). In 228 photos, 30 photos were in Grade 1, 64 photos—Grade 2, 61 photos—Grade 3, 50 photos—Grade 4 and 23 photos—Grade 5. As for FPHL-SI value, the higher GP grade group tended to have a higher FPHL-SI value. The concordance rate for GP evaluation among two or more volunteers and author was 57%, and that between one volunteer and author was 41%, and the concordance rate for photo comparisons, 97% (111/114 cases) of decisions accorded among two or more volunteers and the author, 2% (3/114 cases) of decisions accorded between one volunteer and the author, and 1% of decisions (1/114 cases) did not accord. The incidence rate of hair diameter diversity was well correlated with grades rather than perifollicular pigmentation when compared with dermoscopic features.

The article succeeds in detecting signs of change at an early stage in FPHL using this classification and makes it easier to decide on the treatment protocol and arrests course of FPHL treatment.

Key Messages

- Objective evaluation system of early FPHL to classify early FPHL and also effect of treatment can be achieved with proposed simple system
- If the hair volume is sufficient, the surface reflected light runs parallel keeping a constant distance from the parting and becomes U shape at the whorl—considered a normal state
- No doubt this is a novel idea of classifying FPHL but the fallacies are that one needs to standardize photographs with fixed angle and distance, light adjustment, and background reflection to avoid operator errors. While viewing photographs, observer errors also to be taken into consideration. For practical purposes, this method of classification requires further standardization.

ARTICLE 24

Guidelines for the Diagnosis and Treatment of Male Pattern and Female Pattern Hair Loss, 2017 Version

Manabe M, Tsuboi R, Itami S, et al. Guidelines for the diagnosis and treatment of male-pattern and female-pattern hair loss, 2017 version.
J Dermatol. 2018;45(9):1031-43.

Abstract

A revised version of the 2010 Japanese guidelines aimed at improving further the diagnostic and treatment standards, for both male pattern hair loss (MPHL) and female pattern hair loss (FPHL), has been proposed in this article. Finasteride 1 mg daily, dutasteride 0.5 mg daily and topical 5% minoxidil twice daily for MPHL, and topical 1% minoxidil twice daily for FPHL, as the first-line treatments have been proposed. Adjuvant therapies such as self-hair transplantation, light-emitting diodes and low-level lasers, and also topical application of adenosine for MPHL are being suggested; Prosthetic hair transplantation and oral minoxidil are avoided. Oral finasteride or dutasteride are contraindicated in FPHL. The article also throws light on effectiveness of topical application of t-flavanone, pentadecane, carpronium chloride, cytopurine and ketoconazole, prosthesis such as wig, and also topical application of bimatoprost and latanoprost, and emerging hair regeneration treatments.

COMMENT

The article is a revision of Japanese Dermatological Association's guidelines for the management of androgenetic alopecia 2010. Medline, PubMed, SCI-RUSSCOPUS, Japan Medical Abstracts Society Web and the Cochrane Database of Systematic Reviews, and articles collected by individual members have been assembled to propose the guidelines. Diagnosis of male pattern hair loss (MPHL) and female pattern hair loss (FPHL) is relatively easy, but management is a herculean task. The guidelines are sorted out as a 14 Q—questionnaire format; evidences analyzed accordingly.

- *CQ1:* Is oral administration of finasteride effective? *Recommendation: Strongly recommended for individuals with MPHL, avoided in FPHL.* Oral administration for at least 6 months or more is needed to confirm its effect and its effect is lost once oral administration is discontinued. Grade of recommendation (GOR): A (MPHL), D (FPHL)
- *CQ2:* Is oral administration of dutasteride effective? *Recommendation: Strongly recommended for individuals with MPHL, avoided in FPHL.* Side effects: Reduced libido, impotence and ejaculatory dysfunction. GOR: A (MPHL), D (FPHL)
- *CQ3:* Is topical application of minoxidil effective? *Recommendation: MPHL—5% minoxidil; FPHL—1% minoxidil.* Side

effects: Itching, erythema, desquamation, folliculitis, contact dermatitis and facial hirsutism. GOR: A
- *CQ4*: Is hair transplantation effective? *Self-hair transplantation is strongly recommended for MPHL, permissible in FPHL; but prosthetic hair transplantation is not recommended for MPHL and FPHL.* GOR: B (MPHL) and C1 (FPHL) for self-hair transplantation, and D for prosthetic hair transplantation
- *CQ5*: Is irradiation by light-emitting diodes and low-level lasers effective? *Recommended and also their adverse reactions are relatively mild.* GOR: B
- *CQ6:* Is topical adenosine effective? *Recommended for MPHL; permissible for FPHL.* GOR: B (MPHL), C1 (FPHL)
- *CQ7, 8 and 9*: Is topical carpronium chloride, t-flavanone, cytopurine (CTP), and pentadecane effective? *5% carpronium chloride, 0.1%, 0.3% and 0.5% t-flavanone are permissible, t-flavanone has insufficient evidence in FPHL, and no clinical trials have been conducted of CTP on FPHL; 2.5% pentadecanoic acid glyceride (PDG) also showed moderate improvement, though evidences are insufficient.* GOR: C1
- *CQ10*: Is topical ketoconazole effective? *Permissible in both MPHL and FPHL.* GOR: C1
- *CQ11:* Is use of wigs effective? *Use of a wig does not improve symptoms of hair loss, its use is permissible, when conventional treatments are not successful in improving the symptoms and the QOL is reduced.* GOR: C1
- *CQ12:* Are topical bimatoprost and latanoprost effective? *Not recommended.* GOR: C2
- *CQ13:* Is introduction of growth factors and cell transplantation therapy effective? *Not recommended.* GOR: C2
- *CQ14:* Is oral administration of minoxidil effective? *Not recommended.* Post-marketing survey column lists chest pain, tachycardia, palpitations, breathlessness, dyspnea, congestive heart failure, edema, and weight gain as major side effects. GOR: D.

Key Messages

- *Finasteride 1 mg daily, dutasteride 0.5 mg daily, and topical 5% minoxidil twice daily for MPHL, and topical 1% minoxidil twice daily for FPHL form mainstay*
- *According to American, European, and International Hair Expert Panel for FPHL, it is recommended to use 2% minoxidil twice daily or 5% minoxidil once daily in foam form as against 1% recommended by Japan Dermatology Association. In view of practicality and patient compliance, once daily 5% minoxidil foam or lotion is ideal choice for FPHL which appears to have global consensus.*

ARTICLE 25

Androgenic Alopecia: The Risk-benefit Ratio of Finasteride

Rowland DL, Motofei IG, Păunică I, et al. Androgenic alopecia; the risk–benefit ratio of Finasteride.
J Mind Med Sci. 2018;5(1):1-6.

Abstract

Finasteride is the only FDA-approved systemic therapy available for androgenetic alopecia (AGA). In this article, two perspectives are discussed. Since androgens have important and unique physiological roles within the body, finasteride administration results in androgenic suppression which should be advised with caution. The adverse effects induced by finasteride are neither fully documented nor easily treated. The author feels as alternative therapeutic approaches (such as topical finasteride) become available, the oral administration of finasteride for androgenic alopecia should be re-evaluated.

COMMENT

The person suffering from androgenetic alopecia (AGA) can adapt well to it or can be severely disturbed, the condition being associated with decreased self-esteem, stress, and even depression. Depending on geographic region and culture, bald people are sometimes perceived by others as less attractive and older. This paper presents a series of articles focused on finasteride administration for androgenic alopecia that better evaluate the opportunity of long-term use of an oral chemical compound for a biological condition having nonlife-threatening implications.

Finasteride and dutasteride, inhibitors of the 5α-reductase enzyme, are used in treatment of AGA. Several studies suggest that finasteride should be used with caution for AGA due to the considerable adverse effects induced in some men. These adverse effects are result of action of finasteride in decreasing the conversion of testosterone into the more potent metabolite, dihydrotestosterone (DHT), which plays a critical role in the process of growth and maintenance of several functions of tissues and organs. Thus, inhibitors of 5α-reductase enzyme therefore have the potential to induce a veritable hypogonadal status, yet in turn, the same 5α-reductase inhibitors have the capacity to ameliorate androgenic alopecia.

The authors believe that safety of topical finasteride is much better than systemic finasteride and suggest that *oral* finasteride should be replaced with *topical* administration. Studies have shown that *both scalp and plasma DHT levels significantly decrease after topical application of finasteride, while no changes of testosterone levels were registered in plasma.*

Generally, inhibition of the 5α-reductase enzyme by this drug disrupts the conversion of testosterone to DHT, resulting in a decrease in serum DHT levels by about 65-70%.

The action of the 5α-reductase enzyme is more complex, intervening in the metabolism of multiple neurosteroids within the brain (e.g. testosterone, progesterone, deoxycorticosterone, etc.), neuromodulators that further interfere with cerebral activation of GABA-A receptors. Thus, finasteride leads to several hormonal abnormalities and GABA disruption, with important implications on various neurophysiological processes of the brain. As consequence of cerebral interferences of this drug with sexual neuromodulators and GABA-A receptors, adverse effects described in the case of finasteride can be absent or negligible (anhedonia, lack of mental concentration, insomnia, chronic fatigue, elevated body mass index), or in contrast, quite severe (depression, suicidal ideations, impotence, erectile dysfunction, decreased libido, ejaculation disorders). Such interference is encountered not only during finasteride administration but also after treatment cessation, which is clinically expressed as the post-finasteride syndrome.

Recent studies also suggest that the main (mental and sexual) side effects of finasteride are encountered only in a subset of men, according to structural and informational dichotomies of the brain. Structural dichotomy of the brain results from the lateralization process of the brain, with androgens and female pheromones activating the left hemibrain, and estrogens and male pheromones activating the right hemibrain. According to studies, finasteride adverse effects would be *encountered most strongly in right-handed persons* who present a concrete-thalamic psychophysiologic profile as compared to left-handed persons. *Thus, hand preference and psychological profile/sexual orientation could be used as possible predictive factors for finasteride side effects.*

Thus, there should be risk-benefit ratio in finasteride administration for androgenic alopecia.

Key Messages

- *Finasteride administration places the subjects with androgenic alopecia into an abnormal state, characterized by a low level of DHT. Finasteride adverse effects persist in some men indefinitely after treatment cessation, the corresponding medical support being nonspecific, namely symptomatic*
- *Alternative approach for finasteride administration like topical can be explored*
- *Topical finasteride combined with minoxidil is gaining support as the reports of its efficacy and safety are available; now some reports also evaluated biochemical aspects of topical finasteride suggesting no significant decrease in plasma testosterone levels. The major concern of sexual debility seems to be not an issue with topical finasteride as of now. We need to wait to see the impact of topical finasteride on other aspects of post-finasteride syndrome.*

ARTICLE 26

Medical Comorbidities in Patients with Lichen Planopilaris, A Retrospective Case-control Study

Fertig RM, Hu S, Maddy AJ, et al. Medical comorbidities in patients with lichen planopilaris, a retrospective case-control study.
Int J Dermatol. 2018;57(7):804-9.

Abstract

Lichen planopilaris (LPP) is a chronic inflammatory condition resulting in cicatricial alopecia. The authors have reviewed medical records of 206 LPP [Classical lichen planopilaris (CLPP) and frontal fibrosing alopecia (FFA)] patients to correlate the presence of comorbidities in them. A total of 257 patients of androgenetic alopecia and 66 patients with seborrheic keratosis were used as controls. This study observed higher incidence of systemic lupus erythematosus (SLE) in patients with FFA. Patients with LPP had a lower incidence of diabetes. Patients with CLPP had a lower incidence of hypertension, heart disease and hypothyroidism.

COMMENT

Lichen planopilaris (LPP) is a chronic autoimmune disease. The authors of this article hypothesized that patients with LPP were more likely to have other autoimmune disorders based on the general understanding that LPP is an autoimmune disease. Patients with LPP were more likely to have systemic lupus erythematosus (SLE). As this group of population consisted of only women, it was concluded that women with LPP have an increased risk of SLE. Though SLE causes nonscarring alopecia, this study establishes possible association between SLE and scarring alopecia. Association between single nucleotide polymorphisms of peroxisome proliferator-activated receptor gamma (PPAR-γ) and SLE has been published. Similar studies have suggested that the initial trigger of inflammation in LPP is due to abnormal functioning of the PPAR-γ. Further studies into the association of SLE, LPP and PPAR-γ are required.

Association of hypothyroidism was found to be lower in patients with LPP, which is contradicting to previous published data. Similarly hyperlipidemia, diabetes and hypertension incidences were found to be lower in patients with LPP.

Key Messages
- *Relationship between SLE, LPP, and PPAR-γ is a new arena for further study*
- *There can be a significant association between SLE and LPP in female patients*
- *The study opens up importance of further investigation of efficacious treatment options for SLE in LPP.*

ARTICLE 27

Lichen Planopilaris and Frontal Fibrosing Alopecia as Model Epithelial Stem Cell Diseases

Harries MJ, Jimenez F, Izeta A, et al. Lichen planopilaris and frontal fibrosing alopecia as model epithelial stem cell diseases.
Trends Mol Med. 2018;24(5):435-48.

Abstract

The permanent difficult-to-treat loss of hair is caused due to inflammatory etiology and irreversible damage to immunologically privileged niche of hair follicle (HF) epithelial stem cells (eSCs). We propose that lichen planopilaris (LPP) and frontal fibrosing alopecia (FFA), being the two most common conditions, form excellent model diseases, and easily available human mini-organ, for studying the pathology and biology of adult human eSCs, emphasizing the critical roles for peroxisome proliferator-activated receptor (PPAR)-γ and interferon (IFN)-γ mediated signaling in epithelial–mesenchymal transition (EMT) and immune privilege (IP) collapse of these eSCs, respectively.

COMMENT

Lichen planopilaris (LPP) and frontal fibrosing alopecia (FFA) are inflammatory scalp conditions resulting in permanent alopecia. The central pathogenic processes in both LPP and FFA are epithelial hair follicle stem cells (eHFSCs) depletion and epithelial-mesenchymal transition (EMT) on a background of hair follicles immune privilege collapse predisposing to cytotoxic immune cell attack, eventually resulting in hair follicle (HF) destruction and replacement with fibrous tissue. The authors focus on portraying LPP/FFA as prototypic model of stem cell diseases in which one can explain how human eSCs (epithelial stem cells) are physiologically protected from inflammation-induced damage, and the clinical consequence arising from a failure of these protective mechanisms.

In lesional LPP/FFA HFs, the bulge undergoes major pathological changes such as reduced protein expression of the key bulge stem cell markers K15 and CD200. The niche that surrounds eSCs seems to dictate stem cell behavior and thus primary cicatricial alopecias constitute a great model to dissect the importance of preservation of individual constituents of the local microenvironment for stem cell function. The perifollicular fibrosis is seen may be due to EMT, a process by which epithelial cells lose polarity and cell-to-cell contact and acquire a mesenchymal phenotype. The bulge IP collapse in LPP/FFS shows striking similarities with the bulb immune privilege (IP) collapse seen in alopecia areata (AA). Despite these similarities in immune-pathobiology, the clinical phenotype between LPP/FFA and AA is very different, reflecting the location of the inflammatory attack on key HF structures. To prevent further hair loss treatment for LPP/FFA use nonspecific suppression of the immune system with corticosteroids or other immunosuppressants, to control symptoms and reduce inflammation. Hair regrowth is not possible with medical treatment in LLP/FFA. Hair transplantation is also ineffective since most transplanted HF grafts are destroyed by the inflammatory infiltrate. Potential targets for treatment include using peroxisome proliferator-activated receptor (PPAR)-γ agonists to prevent EMT, and IP-restorative therapies, such as FK506/tacrolimus, to protect eHFSCs from further immune assault.

Little is known about the pathobiology of human eSC niches in extracutaneous tissues, which limits this study.

Lichen planopilaris and FFA provide a disease model for studying the biology and pathology of adult human eSCs in an easily accessible human mini-organ. Emphasizing the critical roles of PPAR-γ and IFN-γ mediated IP collapse and EMT of these eSCs, respectively.

Key Messages

- *Lichen planopilaris and FFA provide excellent model diseases for studying the pathology and biology of adult human eSCs in an easily accessible human mini-organ*
- *Targeting IFN-γ and PPAR-γ mediated signaling by inhibiting the former and stimulating the latter restores both IP collapse and pathological EMT in the bulge*
- *Therapeutically PPAR-γ agonists and tacrolimus are available. Controlled clinical trials are to be initiated.*

ARTICLE 28

Lichen Planopilaris Caused by Wig Attachment: A Case of Koebner Phenomenon in Frontal Fibrosing Alopecia

Taguti P, Dutra H, Trüeb RM. Lichen Planopilaris Caused by Wig Attachment: A Case of Koebner Phenomenon in Frontal Fibrosing Alopecia.
Int J Trichology. 2018;10(4):172-4.

Abstract

Frontal fibrosing alopecia (FFA) represents a distinctive condition with a marginal scarring alopecia along the frontal and temporal hairline. Since its original description, the condition has been recognized to represent a more generalized than localized process, with extension beyond the frontotemporal hairline to include the parieto-occipital hairline and involve peculiar facial papules as evidence of facial vellus hair involvement and loss of peripheral body hair. Finally, the association of FFA with oral lichen planus, nail involvement, and concomitant lichen planopilaris (LPP) points to a close relationship to lichen planus. The Koebner phenomenon or isomorphic reaction has been described in lichen planus, LPP, and ultimately FFA, with face-lift procedures and hair restoration surgery having been implicated as the culprits in the latter. We report the first case of FFA in whom LPP developed at the sites of wig attachments, providing the evidence for Koebner phenomenon. Therefore, wigs are to be included to the list of procedures for hair restoration at risk of eliciting an isomorphic reaction in patients with FFA. Ultimately, the association of Koebner phenomenon with LPP-type lesions in FFA may provide further insight into the underlying pathology and nosology of the condition.

COMMENT

The Koebner phenomenon or isomorphic reaction represents the development of lesions characteristic of a particular disease at the site of a usually physical trauma.

True koebnerization is exhibited by psoriasis, lichen planus and vitiligo.

The Koebner phenomenon has been described in both classic lichen planopilaris (LPP) and frontal fibrosing alopecia (FFA). FFA represents marginal scarring alopecia along the frontal and temporal hairline and eyebrows with histopathological features of LPP.

Besides accidental trauma, elective cutaneous surgical techniques are known to cause koebnerization phenomena, like face-lift procedures and hair restoration surgery on the scalp of susceptible patients.

This case report is of a 59-year-old woman with FFA who developed plaques of scarring alopecia corresponding to LPP, from using a wig.

Patient suffered progressive recession of the frontal hairline and loss of eyebrows since 7 years. Patient had a habit of wearing wig for minimum of 8 hours a day while at work. On removing the wig, five bilateral, symmetrical rounded patches of alopecia in the midline occipital, temporal, and retroauricular regions were observed that corresponded to the sites of fasteners used on the underside of wig. Dermoscopic examination revealed loss of follicular orifices with mild erythema and perifollicular scaling typical for LPP. There was no further evidence of lichen planus of the glabrous skin, the oral mucosa and the nails.

Thus, the patches of scarring alopecia were diagnosed to be of LPP lesions that had developed as a Koebner phenomenon due to pressure of the fasteners imposed when the wig was being worn.

Wig attachments can also elicit an isomorphic reaction in patients with FFA and caution is recommended for surgical interventions during active disease.

Key Messages
⊙ True koebnerization is exhibited by psoriasis, lichen planus and vitiligo
⊙ Besides accidental trauma, elective cutaneous surgical techniques have been implicated in koebnerization phenomena, specifically face-lift procedures and hair restoration surgery on the scalp of susceptible patients in LPP and FFA
⊙ Wig attachments and fasteners are added to the list of procedures for hair restoration that can elicit an isomorphic reaction in patients with LPP and FFA and caution is recommended for surgical interventions during active disease.

ARTICLE 29

Lichen Planopilaris: Retrospective Study on the Characteristics and Treatment of 291 Patients

Babahosseini H, Tavakolpour S, Mahmoudi H, et al. Lichen planopilaris: Retrospective study on the characteristics and treatment of 291 patients.
J Dermatolog Treat. 2018:1-28.

Abstract

Lichen planopilaris (LPP) is an immune-mediated cicatricial alopecia. The main clinical presentations of LPP include classic form, frontal fibrosing alopecia (FFA) and Graham-Little-Piccardi-Lassueur syndrome (GLPLS). We reviewed medical records of all 291 patients diagnosed with LPP from 2006 to 2017 in Department of Dermatology, Tehran University of Medical Sciences. LPP was more common in women than men. Lichen planus (LP) was seen in 59 patients (20.3%). Parietal lesions (69.75%), frontal (27.14%), occipital (23.71%) and temporal (21.64%) were frequently seen in LPP patients. However, trunk hair involvement (15.4% vs. 2.7%; p-value = 0.011) and eyebrow involvement (57.7% vs. 0%; p-value <0.0001) were high in FFA patients. Patients treated with cyclosporine (CSP) achieved partial response (PR) and complete response (CR) faster than with methotrexate (MTX) and mycophenolate mofetil (MMF, p-value = 0.0001). So, CSP and MTX can be considered as effective alternative treatments for nonresponders. Moreover, MTX was more effective than MMF but not different in time to reach PR (p-value = 0.23) or CR (p-value = 0.56). However, CSP and MTX were less safe compared to MMF. The 5α-reductase inhibitors, systemic retinoids (isotretinoin) or their combination were the most effective therapeutic options for FFA patients.

COMMENT

Lichen planopilaris (LPP) is a common primary immune-mediated cicatricial alopecia. It is characterized by selective destruction of the hair follicles by chronic lymphocytic inflammatory process that often results in irreversible scarring alopecia if not treated. This retrospective study included a large number of registered cases of LPP. Characteristics of the disease, the prevalence, comorbidities, clinical features, diagnostic findings, distribution of lesions and symptoms have been defined. The efficacy and safety of different treatments through measuring the response score as well as monitoring patients for several months was done.

The data in this study was collected from 291 patients using a standard questionnaire with clinical data. To assess the disease activity and progression—disease symptoms, perifollicular plugging and positive hair pull test were considered. A therapeutic ladder with topical/intralesional steroid and tacrolimus as first-line, followed by prednisolone, hydroxychloroquine (HCQ), cyclosporine (CSP), and mycophenolate mofetil (MMF) was used. This was followed by methotrexate (MTX), pioglitazone and systemic retinoid. The patients according to their response were divided into three groups—partial response, complete response and nonresponders.

The patients with beard involvement were more prone to refractory disease. More than 50% of the patients needed third-line therapy, and more than 10% of the patients could not achieve complete remission even with several third-line therapies. Frontal fibrosing alopecia (FFA) was treated effectively with 5α-reductase inhibitors and systemic retinoids. CSP and MTX can be considered as effective alternative treatments for nonresponders. The total estimated response rate was 100% for CSP, and the response was seen within a short time from starting.

In this study, the mild disease was treated with first- and second-line drugs, and refractory cases with third-line drugs leading to bias in estimations. The scoring systems of LPP activity index (LPPAI) and FFA-severity index (FFA-SI) were not used in this study due to inclusion of old records. Lack of data in few cases and nonrandomized treatment strategy were its other limitations.

This study explains the demographic data, prevalence, and clinical characters of LPP group of disorders. The treatment mentioned helps in assessing and approaching a patient with LPP in a more strategical and evidence-based manner.

Key Messages

- The continuation of treatment in LPP can decrease the intensity of hair loss and lessen the symptoms even among the partial and nonresponders
- Hydroxychloroquine is often considered as preferred second-line therapy
- Cyclosporine is a potent and fast-acting single agent among the classic LPP patients
- The treatment efficacy and response rates in FFA patients are maximum with 5α-reductase inhibitors and systemic retinoid
- PDE4 inhibitor, apremilast, being reported to be effective in LP. Case-controlled randomized trials on apremilast are awaited.

ARTICLE 30

Premature Graying of Hair: Review with Updates

Kumar AB, Shamim H, Nagaraju U. Premature graying of hair: Review with updates.
Int J Trichol. 2018;10:198-203.

Abstract

This article is a compendium on the premature hair graying (PHG), its causation and treatment options. The underlying pathomechanisms are varied and yet unimpressive to prove direct temporal causation. Premature aging disorders, atopy and autoimmune diseases are significant associations and warrant assessment for syndromes and metabolic diseases. The treatment options are directed for cosmetic concerns essentially; include nutritional supplementation and hair dyes.

COMMENT

Canities (Achromotrichia), when occurs untimely, is termed premature. However, time of onset to define premature hair graying (PHG) in Asians lack data. Clinically, gray hair are coarser, stiffer, and grow faster than pigmented hair. In men, it involve first temples and sideburns; in women, it involves margins of scalp. Early onset and rapid progression are not correlative. PHG should always be differentiated from genetic hypomelanotic disorders (albinism, silvery hair syndrome, Prader-Willi syndrome) and metabolic syndromes (phenylketonuria, histidinemia, oasthouse disease, homocystinuria).

Pathogenesis is still elusive and incomplete. However, proposed possible theories and concrete associations with atopy, autoimmune diseases, do pave way for targeted therapies. Possible theories include—(1) Oxidative stress: Increased reactive oxygen species, absent antioxidants (catalase, methionine sulfoxide reductase), increased pro-oxidants (serum malondialdehyde, whole blood reduced glutathione, serum ferritin), exogenous oxidative damage (UV rays, pollution, alcohol consumption, smoking), stress, and inflammation cause damage to melanocytes leading to gray hair follicles; (2) Premature aging disorders: Progeria and pangeria, have genetic defects in DNA, which are susceptible to damage; (3) Autoimmunity: Autoantibodies targeted at follicular melanocytes as in vitiligo and pernicious anemia; (4) Nutritional deficiencies: Protein–energy malnutrition, deficiency of vitamin B12, vitamin D, copper, iron, calcium, zinc; (5) Endocrinal causes: Decreased thyroid hormones; (6) Drugs: Chemotherapeutic drugs, antimalarials inhibit tyrosine kinase c-kit in melanocytes and hence melanogenesis. Chloroquine reduces pheomelanin production [beware while treating dermatological conditions and rheumatological conditions with hydroxychloroquine sulfate (HCQS)].

The article also elaborates on possible associations of premature canities with other diseases. Increased risk of cardiovascular disease was found by Copenhagen City Heart Study and Aggarwal et al. Another interesting association was with hearing impairment. Conflicting evidence with canities as risk factor for low bone mineral density was also commented upon.

Treating the underlying cause in known cases is the main modality, viz. hormone replacement in hypothyroidism and B12 deficiency. Hair camouflage with natural dyes or synthetic dyes are temporary but also protect from photodamage. Calcium pantothenate 200 mg/day is prescribed often and has yielded satisfactory results only in few instances. Similarly, multivitamins containing zinc, selenium and copper are not promising. P-aminobenzoic acid 200 mg resulted in repigmentation, but is not advocated for sole indication of graying. PUVA therapy and topical prostaglandins (latanoprost used for 3 years yielded results) stimulate melanogenesis.

Strong role of oxidative stress has prompted use of vitamin C, E, green tea extract, selenium, copper, phytoestrogens and melatonin. Plastoquinone (SkQs), a new antioxidant, is being shown to stop age-related changes. Novel concept of topical liposome targeting for molecular strata of proteins, melanin at follicular level, and delivery of drugs through transfollicular route are new in arena.

Key Messages

- *Premature graying of hair needs evaluation to rule out underlying hormonal and nutritional causes, which are treatable*
- *Genetic causes of hypomelanotic hair disorders to be differentiated*
- *Hair dyes are main modality while nutritional supplements are often prescribed*
- *As on date, treatment of idiopathic canities is elusive.*

ARTICLE 31

Association of Epidemiological and Biochemical Factors with Premature Graying of Hair: A Case-control Study

Sharma N, Dogra D. Association of Epidemiological and Biochemical Factors with Premature Graying of Hair: A Case–Control Study.
Int J Trichol. 2018;10:211-7.

Abstract

The article is a cross-sectional case-control study comprised of 120 patients of premature hair graying (PHG) and 120 controls. Epidemiological variables, serum ferritin, serum calcium, serum vitamin D, B12, lipid profile, thyroid profile, and fasting blood sugar were assessed and compared. Atopic diathesis, sedentary lifestyle, positive family history, history of smoking and stress were found to be higher in cases whereas serum calcium, ferritin, vitamin B12, high-density lipoprotein (HDL) cholesterol and high low-density lipoprotein (LDL) cholesterol were lower among cases.

COMMENT

Premature hair graying (PHG) has a strong genetic component possibly dominant pattern of inheritance, compounded with acquired environmental factors, inflammation and psychological stress environmental factors (e.g. UV light and climate), drugs, smoking, deficiency of trace elements and nutritional deficiency, HIV, cystic fibrosis and Hodgkin's lymphoma.

Epidemiological and clinical data on PHG from the Indian subcontinent are lacking. The present study attempts to assess the risk factors associated with PHG; PHG is defined as >5 gray hair in the scalp in patients <25 years of age. A total of 120 cases with PHG and 120 control group comprised age and sex-matched patients. The age of onset, origin, pattern, progression, family history and personal histories such as smoking and alcohol intake were recorded. Biometric data such as height, weight and body mass index were taken. Serum ferritin, calcium, vitamin D and B12, lipid profile, thyroid profile and blood sugar (fasting) were measured in both cases and controls.

Clinically diagnosed PHG were graded into four groups—(1) No gray hair; (2) Mild: <10 gray hair; (3) Moderate: 10-100 gray hair; (4) Severe: >100 gray hair.

The mean age of cases was 15.71 years (M:F—66:54) and of controls was 15.91 years. Majority of the cases were in 11-15 years age group (34.17%). The mean duration of PHG was 21.74 ± 13.86 months (range: 2-60 months), while mean age at onset of graying of hair was 13.80 ± 4.68 years (range: 2-22 years). In cases, the origin of PHG was vertex in 47.50%; frontal in 40%; temporal in 8.33%, and occipital in 4.17% patients and diffuse pattern observed in 95%; 4.17% patients had only frontal involvement and 0.83% only temporal involvement at presentation. Slow progression of PHG was found in 57.50% and rapid in 42.50%. PHG was severe in 38.34%, moderate in 33.33% and mild in 28.33% patients.

Students constituted 79.17%, followed by employees (8.33%), housewives (6.67%) and businessmen (5.83%). Sedentary lifestyle was present in about 22.50% as compared to 7.50% in controls which is statistically highly significant ($p = 0.001$). The younger age of inclusion in the study explains the preponderance of students. About 11.67% of patients were smokers and 0.83% in controls ($p = 0.000$). Smoking causes increased oxidative stress and damage melanocytes. Only 57.50% of patients used hair oil as compared to 31.67% in cases ($p < 0.0001$);

hair oil may be protective in PHG. About 65.83% of patients had positive family history (47.50% parents; 0.83% siblings, and both involved in 17.50%); atopic diathesis seen in 40.83% cases versus 10.83% control (p <0.0001); 65% had normal BMI, underweight (20%), overweight (12.50%), and obese (2.50%).

Perceived stress scale (PSS) was calculated for patients >15 years of age (67 cases and 61 controls) and was significantly higher than average (>16) in 83.59% of patients as compared to 29.51% controls (mean PSS score in cases was 21.20; 13.08 in controls, p <0.0001). Higher PSS score indicates higher emotional stress, which acts as a source of oxidative stress.

Biochemical parameters profile showed that serum calcium was low in 48.33% cases and 25% controls; p = 0.0003, but mean values of serum calcium in both groups were statistically not significant (p = 0.30). Low serum ferritin seen in 48.33% patient versus 20.83% of controls (p <0.0001). Mean value of serum ferritin in cases versus controls was statistically significant (p <0.0001). Iron and calcium affect melanogenesis and so low values suggest their role in PHG. Low serum vitamin D seen in 59.16% patient versus 50% of controls (p = 0.19). Low serum vitamin B12 was seen in 64.17% of cases versus 15% controls (p <0.0001). The mean value of serum vitamin B12 in cases versus controls was also significant (p <0.0001). Vitamin B12 facilitates stabilization of the initial anagen phase of the hair follicle.

Serum LDL levels were significantly raised in cases (21.67%) versus controls (9.17%) (p = 0.01). However, mean serum LDL-cholesterol was 114.72 mg/dL in cases versus 116.42 mg/dL in controls (p = 0.47). About 22.5% of patients had low HDL-C versus 11.67% controls, p = 0.03, which is significant. The mean value of serum HDL-C in cases versus controls, the difference was highly significant (p <0.0001). Presence of dyslipidemia and metabolic risk factors trigger PHG.

Quantification of oxidative stress is vital in substantiating the risk factors and follow-up of patients after correcting the biochemical deficiencies and their effect on PGH definitely validates the compounding factors evaluated in the study.

Key Messages

- The study has looked into many basic aspects of epidemiological and investigational parameters. It is quite interesting that certain facts have been brought into the lime light. However, these following individual factors have to have case-control cross-sectional studies to prove their etiology in PHG
- Family history, atopic diathesis, sedentary lifestyle, smoking, and higher perceived stress found to be associated with PHG
- Low serum calcium, ferritin, vitamin B12, HDL and high LDL point to the need of biochemical profile evaluation in PHG.

ARTICLE 32

Association between Premature Hair Greying and Metabolic Risk Factors: A Cross-sectional Study

Paik SH, Jang S, Joh HK, et al. Association between premature hair greying and metabolic risk factors: a cross-sectional study.
Acta Derm Venereol. 2018;98(8):748-52.

Abstract

The association of hair graying with metabolic syndrome is not well known, while association with obesity and coronary artery disease has been suggested. A cross-sectional study was conducted to identify an association between premature hair graying (PHG) and metabolic risk factors. Of the 1,929 young healthy subjects (1,067 men and 862 women), 704 (36.4%) were categorized in the PHG group. Waist circumference (means of non-PHG vs. PHG, 74.3 vs. 76.3 cm; p <0.001), systolic (109.2 vs. 111.7 mm Hg; p <0.001) and diastolic (65.0 vs. 66.2 mm Hg; p = 0.003) blood pressures, and fasting blood sugar (90.8 vs. 91.6 mg/dL; p = 0.013) were higher and serum high-density lipoprotein (HDL) cholesterol (68.1 vs. 65.4 mg/dL; p <0.001) was lower in PHG group. Multivariate logistic regression analysis showed that metabolic risk factors ≥2 were independently associated with PHG after controlling for confounding factors (odds ratio 1.725; p = 0.036). The present study revealed an association between PHG and metabolic risk factors.

COMMENT

In this study, premature hair graying (PHG) was considered as the presence of gray hair below 30 years of age. The cross-sectional study attempts to determine an association between PHG and metabolic risk factors if any, after adjustment for potential confounders. Epidemiological data regarding known associated risk factors, such as family history of PHG and smoking history, were obtained. Presence and severity of gray hair (grade 0, 0; grade 1, less than 10; grade 2, 10–100; and grade 3, more than 100) was checked. Biochemical and anthropometric parameters related to the metabolic profile were measured and analyzed.

Of the 1,929 participants, 704 (36.4%) were categorized as the PHG group, whereas 1,225 (63.6%), without gray hair, as the non-PHG group. Male sex, family history of PHG, and being overweight were significantly associated with PHG; whereas smoking showed mild association with PHG. In univariate logistic regression analysis, the potential factors for metabolic syndrome components were age, sex, family history of PHG, smoking and metabolic risk factors ≥2. Multivariate logistic regression analysis to identify independent factors associated with PHG, found that a family history of PHG, male sex, metabolic risk factor ≥2, and age were significantly associated with PHG.

Waist circumference, systolic blood pressure (p <0.001), diastolic blood pressure (p = 0.003) and fasting blood sugar were significantly higher and serum high-density lipoprotein (HDL) cholesterol was significantly lower in the PHG group than in the non-PHG group. Prevalence of each metabolic risk factor in PHG and non-PHG groups was evaluated according to adult treatment panel III criteria and found to be higher in PHG group; but statistically insignificant. The prevalence of subjects who had metabolic risk factors ≥2 was also higher in the PHG group than in the non-PHG group.

Total 704 participants with PHG were analyzed regarding the association between the severity of PHG and clinical factors. In the univariate ordinal logistic regression analysis, age, sex, family history of PHG and presence of metabolic risk factor ≥2 were identified as candidate factors with smoking history as a putative candidate factor. In multivariate ordinal logistic regression analysis, family history of PHG, male sex, metabolic risk factor ≥2 and age were significantly associated with the severity of PHG.

The production of endogenous oxidative stress during melanogenesis affects melanocyte stem cells in hair follicles and causes graying. Association of PHG with metabolic risk factors also supports this hypothesis, since they lead to oxidative stress.

The study appears to have limitation as it could not assess the causal relationship and is biased with ethnic study population of Koreans and only early onset PHG is considered. Cross-sectional global studies are required to prove the hypothesis of PHG association with metabolic syndromes.

Key Messages
- *Premature hair graying can be considered as a clinical marker for evaluating patients at risk of metabolic syndrome*
- *Premature hair graying in presence of family history of metabolic syndrome needs evaluations for risk factors as it occurs in early age group.*

ARTICLE 33

Diffuse Scarring Alopecia in a Female Pattern Hair Loss Distribution

Fergie B, Khaira G, Howard V, et al. Diffuse scarring alopecia in a female pattern hair loss distribution. *Australas J Dermatol.* 2018;59(1):e43-6.

Abstract
Three cases of hair loss in a female pattern hair loss (FPHL) distribution with histologic features of lichen planopilaris (LPP) with no characteristic clinical signs of LPP and no histologic features

of FPHL have been described in this case series to highlight scarring alopecia presenting as FPHL, so a clinician needs to be well aware of this possibility especially in a case scenario simulating FPHL, delay in treatment response, and nonresponders.

COMMENT

Three cases of middle-aged Caucasian women presenting with chronic progressive, diffuse hair loss maximally at the frontal and parietal scalp have been described. One patient was on oral antihypertensive and one patient had cervical intraepithelial neoplasia and asthma and was on albuterol inhaler. She was also on ketoconazole 1% shampoo.

On examination, none had perifollicular erythema or hair casts or follicular plugging or follicular ostia.

Biopsy showed superficial interface perifollicular inflammation of lichenoid type with perifollicular fibrosis with normal number of hair follicular units, preserved terminal to vellus ratio, and a normal telogen count which were suggestive of mild lichen planopilaris (LPP).

All patients were treated with topical minoxidil 2% and betamethasone dipropionate lotion 0.5 mg/mL twice daily.

Presence of cicatricial alopecia in a female pattern hair loss (FPHL) distribution lacking perifollicular erythema or follicular hyperkeratosis was unique in the case series. Clinically focal atrichia is specific in cicatricial patterned hair loss (CPHL); however, focal atrichia may be subtle and difficult to discern in pale skin, so biopsy may be required to confirm the diagnosis of a cicatricial alopecia. There remains an overlap in the spectrum of FPHL, CPHL and fibrosing alopecia in a pattern distribution (FAPD). FAPD presents as central scalp scarring hair loss in women or men with underlying established FPHL or male pattern hair loss with perifollicular erythema, follicular hyperkeratosis and loss of follicular orifices and concentric perifollicular lamellar fibrosis, and lymphohistiocytic infiltration in histopathology. However, in frontal fibrosing alopecia (FFA), fronto-temporo-parietal area is involved, though biopsy features are similar to FADP. Diffuse hair loss, lack of perifollicular erythema and perifollicular fibrosis is most consistent with CPHL.

Key Messages

- Scarring alopecia in FPHL distribution with histological features similar to FAPD, but lacking the clinical signs of follicular erythema and hyperkeratosis, is termed a new entity known as cicatricial pattern hair loss
- The article underlines importance of biopsy as the gold standard diagnostic tool in diagnosis and management of all cicatricial alopecias.

ARTICLE 34

Facial Eruptive Vellus Hair Cysts Occurred after 3% Minoxidil Application

Eun DH, Kim SM, Jang YH, et al. Facial Eruptive Vellus Hair Cysts Occurred after 3% Minoxidil Application. *Ann Dermatol. 2018;30(1):95-6.*

Abstract

This article reviews on the rare side effect of minoxidil, which was noted in a 34-year-old patient using 3% minoxidil for longer time. Eruptive vellus hair cyst, a developmental abnormality of vellus hair with no positive family history, was reported after using minoxidil for longer duration.

COMMENT

Minoxidil is a FDA-approved medication for pattern baldness and the main side effect of topical minoxidil is irritant and allergic contact dermatitis due to the presence of propylene glycol as a solvent. Hypertrichosis is also seen due to spreading or individual susceptibility. It has been utilized to treat male and female pattern baldness and alopecia areata multiplex. It is well tolerated when applied but can cause adverse events like irritation, itching, dryness, scaling, telogen shedding and unwanted hair growth. Rare adverse events, which have been reported, are facial swelling, weight gain, chest pain and facial eruptive vellus hair cysts.

This article reports a rare case report of facial eruptive vellus hair cysts caused by the application of 3% minoxidil for the treatment of hair loss. A 34-year-old woman using minoxidil 3% since last 4 years was presented with vellus hair growth on the face mainly over forehead with numerous pinhead-sized papules. She gives history of applying 3% minoxidil since 4 years for hair loss. There was no history of similar complaints in the family members. Eruptive vellus hair cysts remitted after surgical removal, on histopathological examination, laminated keratinous material, and vellus hairs were noted. There were no new lesions after cessation of topical minoxidil.

Eruptive vellus hair cyst is a developmental abnormality of vellus hair follicles caused by the occlusion of infundibulofollicular areas leading to retention of hair, cystic dilatation and atrophy of the hair follicles. It is characterized by asymptomatic follicular papules seen commonly on the chest. The mechanism by which minoxidil causes this vellus is not fully understood but similar side effect is seen with cyclosporine also, which causes hypertrichosis.

Key Messages

- Minoxidil is the most commonly used topical application for AGA. Adverse events (AEs) are common and should all be looked for rare AEs like eruptive vellus hair cyst, which is a developmental abnormality
- There is no association between minoxidil and developmental abnormality of infundibulum, however hypertrichosis might be the cause of cystic changes.

ARTICLE 35

Alopecia in Association with Malignancy: A Review

Suchonwanit P, McMichael AJ. Alopecia in Association with Malignancy: A Review.
Am J Clin Dermatol. 2018;19(6):853-65.

Abstract

Various hair abnormalities can occur in cancer patients due to cancer therapy or paraneoplastic conditions. The mechanisms of these changes are unknown. Alopecia is one of the most common clinical presentations. This review summarizes the clinical characteristics of alopecia that occur in cancer patients and their relationship with the type of malignancy and its treatment.

COMMENT

The clinical characteristics of alopecia, occurring in patients suffering from cancer and its relation with the malignancy type and treatment, have been highlighted in this review. All meta-analyses, randomized clinical trials, cohort studies, review articles, case series and case reports were assessed to include in this review. Hair abnormalities can manifest in diseases of genetic origin that elevate the risk of paraneoplastic syndromes or cancers, and, conversely, due to cancer therapy. Anagen effluvium (AE) and telogen effluvium (TE), alteration of the hair cycle leading to nonscarring hair loss, are important mechanisms leading to malignancy-associated alopecia.

In TE, loss of hair is usually <50% of scalp hair and it happens around 3 months of a triggering event, and is self-limiting within 6–12 months. The cells in hair bulb divide rapidly and are sensitive to cytotoxic substances that impair mitotic and metabolic processes in growing hair follicles. It is severe because 90% of scalp hair are in the anagen phase and this growing hair is shed. In oncology patients, the causative events are administration of chemotherapeutic agents and radiation to the head and neck area.

One of the poor prognostic factors is the occurrence of skin metastases in oncology patients; it may indicate recurrence of remissive malignancy or failure of treatment. Cutaneous metastasis frequently spreads to the scalp. Alopecia neoplastica (AN) refers to alopecia conditions showing hair follicles with direct tumor invasion. In primary alopecia neoplastica, malignancy associated include squamous cell carcinoma, basal cell carcinoma, malignant melanoma, angiosarcoma, extramammary Paget's disease, dermatofibrosarcoma protuberans, cutaneous T cell lymphoma and hemangioendothelioma. Metastatic breast cancer is the most common association seen in secondary alopecia neoplastica. AN usually presents as multiple or single areas of hair loss, with size ranging from 2 cm^2 to 20 cm^2. It presents as plaques, patches, papules, cystic lesions, nodules, ulcerated lesions and sclerodermoid lesions or telangiectatic lesions. The histopathology of AN reveals features consistent with primary malignancy in dermis or subcutaneous stroma with infiltration of neoplastic cells, and in association with decreased number of pilosebaceous unit and hair follicle miniaturization. Early detection and early treatment can be done by identification of underlying metastatic malignancy.

Malignancy management-related alopecias are hair loss conditions that are seen with treatment of cancer such as radiation and chemotherapy. Hair loss usually initiates 7–14 days following exposure to precipitating factor and reduces by 1–2 months. It also depends on the schedule and the dose of chemotherapy. Degree of follicular damage from chemotherapy was hypothesized to be due to p53-dependent apoptosis of hair matrix cells. CIA may occur with different manifestations, such as TE and AE due to administration of chemotherapeutic agents, or alopecia associated with biologic agents. Several chemotherapeutic agents cause AE including alkylating agents, antimicrotubule agents, antimetabolites and topoisomerase inhibitors. Specialized forms of CIA have been reported in various novel anticancer treatments. Neoadjuvant endocrine therapies, such as selective estrogen receptor modulators and aromatase inhibitors, have been reported to cause nonscarring alopecia in an androgenetic pattern. Alopecia areata (AA) has been reported in association with immune checkpoint and interferon-α inhibitors. Patients receiving EGFRIs have experienced scarring alopecia, which manifested as tufted folliculitis or erosive pustular dermatosis. Permanent CIA is a type of hair loss, following chemotherapy with no or incomplete hair regrowth within 6 months. RIA refers to AE caused by radiation treatment due to acute damage of actively dividing matrix cells. By 2–4 months, complete hair regrowth generally occurs. It can be permanent or reversible.

Paraneoplastic alopecia is a group of nongenetic, nonsyndromic hair loss conditions that are seen in along with malignancy. The paraneoplastic alopecias are AA, TE, nonspecific scarring alopecia and alopecia mucinosa. AA is associated with hematological malignancies. Alopecia mucinosa is associated with mycosis fungoides. Nonspecific scarring alopecia is seen in association with multiple myeloma.

Early detection and management of alopecia in malignancy can improve quality of life and morbidity in affected patients.

Key Messages

- Alopecia is one of the common clinical presentations in oncology patients
- Clinicians have to distinguish telogen hair from anagen hair in CIA and alopecia neoplastica as it has therapeutic and prognostic implications. Trichoscopy aids in assisting clinical diagnosis
- Alopecia in association with malignancy can be classified based on etiology into alopecia neoplastica, malignancy treatment-related alopecia and paraneoplastic alopecia
- Alopecia may reflect the status of underlying malignancy.

ARTICLE 36

Incidence and Risk Factors for Alopecia in Survivors of Critical Illness: A Multi-centre Observational Study

Battle CE, Lynch C, Thorpe C, et al. Incidence and risk factors for alopecia in survivors of critical illness: A multi-centre observational study.
J Crit Care. 2019;50:31-5.

Abstract

This is a multicenter observational study in 10 intensive care units (ICUs) that investigated the incidence, nature and risk factors for patient-reported alopecia in survivors of critical illness in a predesigned survey post 3 months ICU discharge. Out of 123 patients who completed survey, 44 had alopecia and the only risk factor was sepsis/septic shock. This highlights the need for evaluation of alopecia in survivors of critical illness, who had sepsis/septic shock.

COMMENT

During recovery from acute critical illness phase, alopecia can prove distressing for the patient. Various types of alopecia occur in critically ill patients including telogen effluvium, pressure alopecia and traction alopecia. This study was done to investigate the incidence, nature and risk factors for patient-reported alopecia in a cohort of critical illness survivors.

This multicentric study included patients in ICU of 10 hospitals in Wales with 3 months follow-up. Medical and surgical specialties were included and burn and pediatric specialties were excluded. Those who had an

ICU stay of more than 5 days were included. At 3 months post-ICU discharge, a predesigned survey was sent to each participant, with a follow-up phone call for completion, if the survey was not returned.

The nonresponders were found to be significantly younger than the responders and most were males. A sudden onset of alopecia was reported in 11 (25%). The only risk factor for alopecia in survivors of critical illness was a diagnosis of sepsis/septic shock. This reflects the reduction in tissue perfusion which occurs in sepsis but interestingly serum lactate did not differ significantly between the two groups, nor did the APACHE II illness severity score predict the development of alopecia. The most common type of hair loss reported in this study was all over thinning, ranging from minor to severe, starting within the 1st month following ICU discharge.

Further research is required to recognize the pathophysiological processes of sepsis/septic shock that seem to be causing alopecia in this patient population. Due to the distressing nature of the condition, the potential for alopecia to occur in the recovery phase of critical illness should be communicated more widely with patients and their relatives, especially when sepsis has been identified.

Key Messages

- *Various types of alopecia occur in critically ill patients including telogen effluvium, pressure alopecia and traction alopecia*
- *Septic shock is one of the risk factors for alopecia in survivors of critical illness*
- *This is a novel study which can be replicated in many multispecialty hospitals having ICU facilities. The impact of alopecia on lifestyle is huge, given the cause of hair loss*
- *Communications and reassurance in postrecovery period are crucial part of counseling in these patients.*

Section 3 Therapeutic Trichology (Medical)

ARTICLE 37

Controversies in the Treatment of Androgenetic Alopecia: The History of Finasteride

Andy G, John M, Mirna S, et al. Controversies in the treatment of androgenetic alopecia: The history of finasteride. *Dermatol Ther. 2019;32(2):e12647.*

Abstract

Presently, for male androgenetic alopecia (AGA), Food and Drug Administration (FDA) approved treatment options are minoxidil and finasteride. The response of minoxidil is seen in less than 40% of men even after 24 weeks of treatment. In contrast, finasteride works in more than 80% of men after 12 months of therapy. The perception of drug has changed recently due to controversial adverse sexual side effect profile.

COMMENT

This article analyses the controversy surrounding the finasteride induced sexual side effects.

In 1992, the United States Food and Drug Administration (USFDA) approved finasteride 5 mg daily for the treatment of benign prostatic hyperplasia (BPH). Proscar Long-term Efficacy and Safety Study (PLESS), a 4-year placebo-controlled study of 3,040 men suffering from BPH was conducted (USFDA, 2011). It showed that during 1st year, side effects like decreased libido and erectile dysfunction were more in finasteride group as compared to placebo group. However, in the 2nd year of the study, there was no significant difference in the rate of sexual adverse events between the finasteride and placebo groups.

Subsequently low-dose finasteride 1 mg was approved by USFDA in 1997 for male androgenetic alopecia (AGA).

In a study period of 12 months, 945 subjects were administered finasteride 1 mg and 934 subjects were administered a placebo. During the 1st year, decreased libido was reported in 1.8% of subjects in the finasteride group versus 1.3% in the placebo group. Erectile dysfunction was reported in 1.3% of subjects in the finasteride group versus 0.7% in the placebo group. In the 5th year of treatment, the rate of adverse events decreased to less than 0.3% in all groups (USFDA, 2011). Additionally, men that discontinued therapy had no further sexual adverse events. A recent study by Gupta et al. by examining Food and Drug Administration Adverse Event Reporting System (FAERS) database found that occurrence of sexual adverse events from finasteride is rare.

In 2011, the USFDA conducted a post marketing evaluation of reported cases of persistent sexual dysfunction after finasteride discontinuation. About 2,527 cases, the USFDA came across 59 reported cases of sexual dysfunction where it lasted for 3 or more months after finasteride discontinuation. Out of them, 20 cases had sexual dysfunction lasting 1-2 years and 7 had for more than 3 years. It was noted that in some of the cases subjects had low testosterone values. After which Merck has modified finasteride (Propecia) label to disclose the post marketing sexual adverse events. Shortly after Merck revised its label, thousands of websites claimed that Propecia and finasteride cause erectile dysfunction and loss of libido. This has changed the perception of finasteride as causing serious sexual side effects. The low levels of testosterone are associated with erectile dysfunction, decreased libido and depression.

It is recognized that males experience a gradual decline in testosterone concentration starting as early as their third decade, but erectile dysfunction can affect men in any age group. It was observed that sexual dysfunction in patients with finasteride have same rate of occurrence in general population. Moreover, the age of onset for hormonal changes that manifest as sexual dysfunction often coincide with the age of onset for the development of AGA. Thus, the patients having AGA have more chances of experiencing sexual dysfunction. Hence, it may be difficult to attribute the development of sexual dysfunction to finasteride use alone.

The other drugs used frequently like selective serotonin reuptake inhibitors (SSRIs) and serotonin norepinephrine reuptake inhibitors (SNRIs) are well known for their sexual side effects. SSRIs have shown higher rate of sexual dysfunction in over 50% subjects compared to finasteride in less than 1%.

The author suggests screening of patients with a questionnaire to identify the subjects who are likely to develop sexual dysfunction. Also he recommends that we should give an informed choice to candidate who is fit for finasteride by explaining the evidence from the controlled studies presented on the finasteride FDA label.

In the era of internet savvy patients and increased incidence of medicolegal issues, clinicians should be able to convey patients the possible adverse events before prescribing finasteride and choice better left to patients. This does not mean we should be afraid of prescribing finasteride. Always counsel the patients on pros and cons of therapy and benefits of finasteride therapy has to be offered to the deserving patients

Key Messages

- *Finasteride is the only FDA approved oral drug which has consistent efficacy to arrest the progression of AGA*
- *The rate of sexual side effects associated with finasteride has same prevalence as in general population*
- *The prescribing doctor should screen the patient with a questionnaire to identify patients who have more potential for developing side effects and can avoid finasteride in them.*

ARTICLE 38

Adverse Effects with Finasteride 5 mg/day for Patterned Hair Loss in Premenopausal Women

Oliveira-Soares R, André MC, Peres-Correia M. Adverse effects with finasteride 5 mg/day for patterned hair loss in premenopausal women.
Int J Trichology. 2018;10(1):48-50.

Abstract

Finasteride 5 mg/day had been used in female patterned hair loss (FPHL) in both pre- and post-menopausal women with good success. In this study, side effects associated with finasteride in premenopausal women are studied.

COMMENT

This study highlights the side effects of finasteride 5 mg/day used in premenopausal women (18 years old or more). From 336 patients with female patterned hair loss (FPHL) asked to be enrolled in the study, only 256 patients were included with the diagnosis of FPHL and without treatment for the previous 6 months or having stopped treatment for 6 months.

Finasteride was given in dose of 5 mg/day with informed consent. The adverse effects were assessed by patient enquiry and blood tests at 3, 6, 12, 18, 24 and 36 months. A pretreatment blood test was obtained at day 0.

Safety evaluation was done at 0, 3, 6, 12 and 18 months by asking for symptoms and blood test (blood count, liver enzymes, total bilirubin, glycemia, urea, creatinine, total testosterone, free testosterone, dehydroepiandrosterone sulfate (DHEAS), delta-4 androstenedione, 5α-dihydrotestosterone, 17-beta-hydroxyprogesterone, cortisol, prolactin, luteinizing hormone and follicle-stimulating hormone).

The observation suggested that 1 in 5 patients have reported adverse effect at first visit at 3 months. Most of the adverse effects decreased or disappeared with time. Only 1 in 30 patients has adverse effects at the last observation, 36th month.

The most common adverse effects were libido reduction, mastalgia or hypertrichosis/hirsutism, headache which decrease over time.

The study concluded that finasteride is not only more effective in premenopausal women but also adverse effects are much more common, especially in the first months of the treatment. But these adverse effects decrease over time, reason being some adaptive hormonal changes in hypophysis/gonadal axis or in brain perception.

Key Messages

- Finasteride 5 mg/day has good efficacy in treatment of FPHL in women of premenopausal age group with adverse effects common in first 3 months which decrease with continuous use
- Finasteride therapy in premenopausal women should be used with caution and preferably with oral contraception to prevent accidental pregnancies as finasteride is category X drug.

ARTICLE 39

'Post-Finasteride Syndrome': What to Tell Our Female Patients?

Mervis JS, Borda LJ, Miteva M. 'Post-finasteride syndrome': What to tell our female patients?
Br J Dermatol. 2018;179(3):785-6.

Abstract

This article analyses frequency of Post-Finasteride syndrome (PFS) in female patients receiving finasteride. Literature analysis from published data showed that PFS incidence in female is insignificant.

COMMENT

Post-Finasteride syndrome (PFS) is a controversial entity in men taking finasteride for androgenetic alopecia (AGA). "Post-finasteride syndrome" is a collective term which includes not only the sexual side effects like decreased libido, erectile and ejaculatory dysfunction, and gynecomastia, but also depression, cognitive impairment, fatigue and suicidal ideation, which are supposed to be related to finasteride use that may persist or commence after discontinuation of the drug. The various reasons mentioned in literature include decreased production of neurosteroids, impaired testosterone metabolism, leading to relative estrogen excess.

Though not approved, finasteride is being used in female pattern hair loss (FPHL). However literature on PFS in females is lacking. This research letter aims at evaluating the frequency of reported side effects of finasteride use, including PFS, in women. The authors collected data from articles from Pubmed and they found that prevalence of adverse effects, including decreased libido was very low and data on PFS among women taking finasteride for hair loss was not available. Though loss of libido and sexual dysfunction has been reported in few studies, it is unclear if it is drug induced or may be attributed to normal physiological changes.

Key Messages

- Post-Finasteride syndrome, apart from sexual dysfunction, also includes psychiatric symptoms
- Though PFS is more commonly reported in males on finasteride, its incidence in female patients is insignificant.

ARTICLE 40

Female Pattern Hair Loss: A Pilot Study Investigating Combination Therapy with Low-dose Oral Minoxidil and Spironolactone

Sinclair RD. Female pattern hair loss: a pilot study investigating combination therapy with low-dose oral minoxidil and spironolactone.
Int J Dermatol. 2018;57(1):104-9.

Abstract

Background: The oral antihypertensives, minoxidil and spironolactone, are known to stimulate hair growth.

Objective: To report on a case series of pattern hair loss (PHL) in female patients treated with once daily spironolactone 25 mg and minoxidil 0.25 mg.

Methods: Women newly diagnosed with a stage 2–5 PHL according to Sinclair classification were scored for hair density and hair shedding before and after 12 months of treatment with oral spironolactone 25 mg and minoxidil 0.25 mg.

Results: This observational pilot study included a total of 100 women. Mean age was 48.44 years (range 18–80). Sinclair 2.79 (range 2–5) and 4.82 was mean hair loss severity score and mean hair shedding score at baseline, respectively. Mean diagnosis duration was 6.5 years (range 0.5–30). Mean hair loss reduction severity score was 0.85 at 6 months and 1.3 at 12 months. Mean hair shedding reduction score was 2.3 at 6 months and 2.6 at 12 months. Mean blood pressure change was 6.48 mm Hg diastolic and 4.52 mm Hg systolic. Mild side effects were seen in eight women. Hyperkalemia or any other blood test abnormality were not seen in any patients. Two women who developed urticaria discontinued treatment, but six of these women continued treatment.

Limitations: Open-label observational, uncontrolled and prospective study.

Discussion: Once daily capsules containing spironolactone 25 mg and minoxidil 0.25 mg appear to be effective and safe in the treatment of female pattern hair loss (FPHL). Further, placebo-controlled studies to investigate this further are needed.

COMMENT

Female pattern hair loss (FPHL) is a complex polygenic disorder characterized clinically by diffuse hair thinning over the midfrontal scalp and increased hair shedding. When applied topically, minoxidil has been shown to arrest hair loss or to induce mild-to-moderate hair regrowth in approximately 60% of women with FPHL. Spironolactone is widely used off-label in the treatment of FPHL. The authors aim to study the safety and usefulness of a single, once daily low-dose oral minoxidil in combination with spironolactone in the treatment of FPHL.

100 women with a Sinclair stage 2–5 FPHL were considered and reviewed at 3 monthly intervals. They were treated with a once daily capsule containing minoxidil 0.25 mg and spironolactone 25 mg and followed prospectively for 12 months.

The combination of spironolactone and minoxidil is likely to have an additive benefit in FPHL. The side effects of hyperkalemia, creatinine elevation and hepatitis reported with spironolactone, were not encountered at the dose used in this study.

The study is limited by being a prospective, uncontrolled and open-label observational study.

Most women noticed a reduction in hair shedding at 3 months and an increase in hair density at 6 months. Hence, low-dose oral minoxidil was well tolerated in the majority of patients with FPHL and is a reasonable alternative in women intolerant of or unwilling to use topical minoxidil.

Key Messages

- Once daily capsules containing minoxidil 0.25 mg and spironolactone 25 mg appear to be safe and effective in the treatment of FPHL
- The combination of spironolactone and minoxidil is likely to have an additive benefit in FPHL
- This appears to be an interesting study that opens up new avenue for treatment of FPHL. We need to wait and see if oral minoxidil alone works.

ARTICLE 41

Clinical Efficacy of Oral Administration of Finasteride at a Dose of 2.5 mg/day in Women with Female Pattern Hair Loss

Won YY, Lew BL, Sim WY. Clinical efficacy of oral administration of finasteride at a dose of 2.5 mg/day in women with female pattern hair loss.
Dermatol Ther. 2018;31(2):e12588.

Abstract

This study was done to evaluate the effectiveness of oral finasteride in females who were suffering from hair loss which presents as diffuse thinning over the mid-frontal scalp. A total of 544 premenopausal or postmenopausal patients with female pattern hair loss (FPHL) were retrospectively investigated who were given finasteride at a daily dosing of 2.5 mg. The exclusion criteria were patients with a follow-up period of less than 3 months as well as those patients who were prescribed other FPHL treatment modalities such as topical minoxidil. About 112 patients were assessed based on their medical records and clinical photographs. The evaluation was done using the Ludwig scale during their initial visit. Out of the 112 patients, 59 patients were categorically placed in grade I, 47 patients in grade II, and 6 in grade III. Out of the 112 patients, 33 showed slight improvement, 73 patients showed significant improvement, while the remaining 6 had no improvement. Thus it was concluded that finasteride had a better effect on hair growth in patients who demonstrated a lower Ludwig score and an older age of onset.

COMMENT

Female pattern hair loss (FPHL) has diffuse thinning in the center with maintenance of the frontal hair line. Different treatment modalities including use of topical minoxidil, oral anti-androgen agents, and 5α-reductase inhibitors including finasteride and dutasteride have been tried as treatment for FPHL. Finasteride is a competitive and specific inhibitor of type II 5α-reductase and prevents the conversion of testosterone to dihydrotestosterone (DHT); the latter is known to play a role in causing hair follicle miniaturization. The recommended dose of oral finasteride is 1 mg/day in male androgenetic alopecia (AGA). Studies in females showed 1 mg/day of finasteride to be ineffective and 5 mg/day was found to be effective but with several adverse effects. So this study evaluated retrospectively, 2.5 mg/day of finasteride daily in a large sample size. All postmenopausal and premenopausal women not planning to get pregnant were included in this study. Global photographs were used to evaluate efficacy.

In this study, most premenopausal or postmenopausal patients with FPHL who had been treated >3 months responded to 2.5 mg/day of finasteride. It was well accepted by patients without any adverse effects. It was observed that finasteride showed a good response with longer duration of treatment. A positive correlation was demonstrated between the age of onset of this condition and improvement in hair growth. Patients with Ludwig grade I showed a higher mean score of improvement than those with Ludwig grade II and III.

Though the sample size of this study was large, the limitations were that it was a retrospective study and no phototrichogram was used to evaluate changes in the hair thickness. This study concluded that use of finasteride at a dose of 2.5 mg daily for FPHL achieves the same safety and efficacy as a daily dose of 5 mg of this drug.

Key Messages

- Finasteride is a competitive and specific inhibitor of type II 5α-reductase and prevents the conversion of testosterone to DHT which is responsible for hair follicle miniaturization
- Finasteride in the dose of 2.5 mg/day given for more than 3 months gives a good response in FPHL and is better tolerated
- Note that there is a paucity of head to head comparison of 2.5 mg versus 5 mg finasteride in FPHL, but most of studies recently published advocate 2.5 mg/day of finasteride in FPHL.

ARTICLE 42

Case Series of Oral Minoxidil for Androgenetic and Traction Alopecia: Tolerability and the Five C's of Oral Therapy

Beach RA. Case series of oral minoxidil for androgenetic and traction alopecia: Tolerability & the five C's of oral therapy. *Dermatol Ther. 2018;31(6):e12707.*

Abstract

Topical minoxidil is an effective, FDA-approved treatment for androgenetic alopecia (AGA) and has also been shown to help traction alopecia (TA). A total of 20 patients, 16 AGA patients and 4 TA patients, received 3 months course of 1.25 mg of oral minoxidil. This report deduces 5 C's of oral minoxidil as Convenient to swallow, Cosmesis, Cost-savings, Co-therapy and good Compliance.

COMMENT

Topical minoxidil is an effective, FDA-approved treatment for androgenetic alopecia (AGA) and has also been shown to help traction alopecia (TA).

Orally, minoxidil is prescribed as an antihypertensive with potential cardiac side effects such as edema, pericarditis, or pericardial effusion. Approximately 80% of users develop hypertrichosis with elongation and thickening of hair at various sites including the scalp.

The potential cardiovascular effects may discourage its prescription for hair loss by dermatologists. This case series details the tolerability and adherence rates of oral minoxidil for treatment of AGA or TA.

Twenty patients (18 women and 2 men) diagnosed with AGA (16 patients) and TA (four patients) were prescribed 3 months course of 1.25 mg of oral minoxidil. This dose was determined after reviewing reports of successful hair growth with 1 mg dosing, and based on the availability of a 2.5 mg tablet which was halved. The medication was continued by 14 patients at the end of study.

Thirty-three percent patients (6/8 patients) reported reduced hair shedding, while 28% (5/8 patients) reported enhanced scalp hair. About 39% (7/18) reported hypertrichosis over the face (most common, around lip) and arms, yet all the affected continued treatment due to its perceived benefit for hair over their scalp.

In all patients, blood pressure (BP) monitoring was done. Among nine patients who monitored their BP, in seven patients it remained within normal range and in two patients it improved from hypertensive levels. One patient (6%) reported symptoms of hypotension and urticaria for around 8–10 days. Significant cardiac morbidity was not experienced in any patients.

This report deduces 5 C's of oral minoxidil—*Convenient* to swallow oral minoxidil than topical application. This is especially for those patients who do not prefer to wet their hair on daily basis.

The oral therapy did not generate product residue or distort gray hair, hence, patients noted enhanced *Cosmesis*.

Cost-savings was attained by supply of oral minoxidil for 3 months relative to the topical over-the-counter (OTC) product.

Without the use of competing topical minoxidil, it was simpler to visually enhance fullness by *Co-therapy* with application of commercial keratin fibers.

Good *Compliance* was demonstrated by 78% of patients, who continued oral therapy till last follow-up.

The therapeutic benefit of oral minoxidil, as indicated by recent reports, further requires subsequent investigations that objectively measure hair growth over the scalp and help in establishing optimal dosage of oral minoxidil.

Key Messages

- *Despite well-established to treat hair loss and enhance hair growth, the efficacy and safety of oral minoxidil for treatment of AGA has not been evaluated*
- *This case series details the tolerability and adherence rates of oral minoxidil and the benefits over topical minoxidil*
- *Convenience, cosmesis, co-therapy, cost savings and compliance are found to be the advantages of oral minoxidil with a good safety profile.*

ARTICLE 43

An Open-label Randomized Multicenter Study Assessing the Noninferiority of a Caffeine-based Topical Liquid 0.2% versus Minoxidil 5% Solution in Male Androgenetic Alopecia

Dhurat R, Chitallia J, May TW, et al. An open-label randomized multicenter study assessing the noninferiority of a caffeine-based topical liquid 0.2% versus minoxidil 5% solution in male androgenetic alopecia.
Skin Pharmacol Physiol. 2017;30(6):298-305.

Abstract

The article analyzes if a caffeine-based 0.2% topical liquid is no less effective in comparison with minoxidil 5% solution in the treatment of androgenetic alopecia (AGA) in males (n = 210). The primary end point was kept as the percentage change in the proportion of anagen hair at baseline and at 6 months which were analyzed using trichogram in frontal and occipital area. The article hypothesizes that a caffeine-based 0.2% topical liquid is not inferior to minoxidil 5% solution in the treatment of AGA in males.

COMMENT

Androgenetic alopecia (AGA) is the most common hair problem encountered in trichology clinics. Apart from FDA approved topical therapy with minoxidil, many other non-minoxidil solutions are available. One such topical therapy is caffeine-based solution. Caffeine, being a phosphodiesterase inhibitor, increases cyclic adenosine monophosphate levels in cells and consequently promotes cell proliferation through stimulating cell metabolism. This mechanism counteracts the testosterone/dihydrotestosterone-induced miniaturization of the hair follicle. Caffeine in shampoo formulation has also shown penetration into hair follicle.

In this prospective randomized controlled study, the authors have compared the caffeine-based topical 0.2% liquid as against 5% minoxidil solution. This study showed that caffeine based liquid to be as effective as minoxidil at 6 months, which was assessed using the anagen rate in occipital and frontal trichogram, which was done in two groups: per-protocol (PP) and intention-to-treat (ITT) population.

This study showed noninferiority of caffeine as compared to 5% minoxidil solution in males with AGA. The adverse effect profile assessed in this study concluded, both the solutions to be well tolerated and minimal AE was seen in minoxidil group but not in caffeine group.

This study was limited by having a broad inclusion criteria and being an open-label design which would lead to unintentional bias.

The study concluded that naturally occurring ingredients like caffeine can be considered as an effective alternative in hair loss management.

> **Key Messages**
> - The efficacy of caffeine-based preparation is no less than minoxidil in the management of AGA
> - Caffeine is a phosphodiesterase inhibitor and counteracts the testosterone/dihydrotestosterone-induced miniaturization of the hair follicle
> - Topical caffeine-based liquids and shampoos are available for the treatment of hair loss but lack structured case control randomized studies. The evidence for caffeine in AGA treatments is coming as case reports and individual experiences. This study is the first attempt to compare with minoxidil. As of now, formulation of caffeine can be regarded as adjunctive and reserved for minoxidil intolerant patients.

ARTICLE 44

Minoxidil in the Treatment of Androgenetic Alopecia

Goren A, Naccarato T. Minoxidil in the treatment of androgenetic alopecia.
Dermatol Ther. 2018;31(5):e12686.

Abstract

In United States, approximately 30 million women and 50 million men suffer from androgenetic alopecia (AGA; also known as pattern hair loss), as estimated by the National Institutes of Health (US NIH, 2018). Only topical drug for the treatment of both male and female pattern hair loss (FPHL) is minoxidil. In the US, a maximum concentration of 5% of minoxidil is approved for over-the-counter (OTC). In this article, we summarize the novel developments and recent discoveries in the use of minoxidil, as well as the findings of the pivotal studies used in support of the drug's approval for the treatment of AGA.

COMMENT

According to the National Institutes of Health (NIH), there are approximately 50 million men and 30 million women suffering from androgenetic alopecia (AGA) in United States. Currently, there are only two FDA approved drugs for the treatment of AGA: oral finasteride and topical minoxidil. This review article aims at reviewing important developments in the treatment and diagnosis of AGA.

The majority of men respond to finasteride, by inhibiting the conversion of testosterone to dihydrotestosterone; however, recently, several cases of irreversible sexual adverse events associated with the use of finasteride are being reported. Subsequently, the number of finasteride prescriptions for AGA has declined significantly.

Minoxidil is approved over-the-counter (OTC) drug at a maximum concentration of 5% in the United States. Minoxidil is a prodrug converted to its active form, minoxidil sulfate, by the sulfotransferase enzyme expressed in the outer root sheath of hair follicles. While topical minoxidil has an excellent safety record, the efficacy of the drug remains low. The sulfotransferase enzymatic activity in plucked hair follicles predicts a patient's response to topical minoxidil. According to few reports, the sulfotransferase enzymatic assay was able to accurately identify 94% of nonresponders to topical minoxidil. Female pattern hair loss (FPHL) patients were identified as nonresponders to 5% topical minoxidil in few studies. Low minoxidil metabolizer is unlikely to respond to low dosage of minoxidil nor experience cardiac adverse events at higher dosages. Salicylic acid is known to inhibit $SULT1A1$ enzyme expression in the liver; thus, it is of clinical significance to understand the effect of daily aspirin use on minoxidil response in hair follicles.

Further studies aim to develop a new higher concentration topical minoxidil formula (up to 15%) for nonresponders to 5% topical minoxidil identified by sulfotransferase enzymatic assay.

Key Messages

- Several cases of irreversible sexual adverse events associated with the use of finasteride are being reported
- The sulfotransferase enzymatic activity in plucked hair follicles predicts a patient's response to topical minoxidil
- The response rate of minoxidil uses opens up a new arena of increasing dose of minoxidil probably in a clinical scenario where estimation of sulfotransferase enzyme is not possible but potential for high concentration of minoxidil is available, then a therapeutic trial can be given
- Estimation of sulfotransferase enzyme activity in plucked hair follicles is a valuable tool in predicting response to minoxidil.

ARTICLE 45

Oleic Acid Nanovesicles of Minoxidil for Enhanced Follicular Delivery

Kumar P, Singh SK, Handa V, et al. Oleic Acid Nanovesicles of Minoxidil for Enhanced Follicular Delivery. *Medicines (Basel). 2018;5(3):103*

Abstract

Current topical minoxidil (MXD) formulations involve an unpleasant organic solvent which causes patient incompliance in addition to side effects in some cases. Therefore, the objective of this work was to develop an MXD formulation providing enhanced follicular delivery and reduced side effects. Oleic acid (OA), being a safer material, was utilized to prepare the nanovesicles, which were characterized for size, entrapment efficiency (EE), polydispersity index (PDI), zeta potential and morphology. The nanovesicles were incorporated into the emugel Sepineo® P 600 (2% w/v) to provide better longer contact time with the scalp and improve physical stability. The formulation was evaluated for in vitro drug release, ex vivo drug permeation and drug deposition studies. Follicular deposition of the vesicles was also evaluated using a differential tape stripping technique and elucidated using confocal microscopy. The optimum oleic acid vesicles (OAVs) measured particle size was 317 ± 4 nm, with high EE ($69.08 \pm 3.07\%$), narrow PDI (0.203 ± 0.01), and a negative zeta potential of -13.97 ± 0.451. The in vitro drug release showed the sustained release of MXD from vesicular gel. The skin permeation and deposition studies revealed superiority of the prepared MXD vesicular gel (0.2%) in terms of MXD deposition in the stratum corneum (SC) and remaining skin over MXD lotion (2%), with enhancement ratios of 3.0 and 4.0, respectively. The follicular deposition of MXD was 10-fold higher for vesicular gel than the control. Confocal microscopy also confirmed the higher absorption of rhodamine via vesicular gel into hair follicles as compared to the control. Overall, the current findings demonstrate the potential of OAVs for effective targeted skin and follicular delivery of MXD.

COMMENT

Minoxidil (MXD) and finasteride are the only Food and Drug Administration approved topical agents for the treatment of hair loss. The percutaneous absorption of the drug has been limited by stratum corneum (SC). Organic solvents have been added to MXD containing current products to increase the solubility and penetration of the drug, but it leads to poor patient compliance. Oleic acid vesicles (OAVs) have previously shown to increase absorption of the drug through the skin. It has been used as a carrier for topical administration of many drugs. The ideal formulation to target hair follicle should involve a composition and physical property which can facilitate fusion of fatty acid in sebum. This makes fatty acid vesicles an attractive delivery system for targeted drug delivery to the hair follicles.

In this study, ex vivo skin permeation and deposition of self-assembled nanovesicles of oleic acid (OA) and phosphatidylcholine were conducted to determine the drug accumulation in different layers of skin using confocal laser scanning microscopy (CLSM). The formulation was evaluated for in vitro drug release, ex vivo drug permeation, and drug deposition studies.

The finalized formulation (OAV1) in this study consisted of three parts of fatty acid and one part of phosphatidylcholine. As OA concentration increased, vesicle size also increased while entrapment efficiency (EE) decreased. Increase in the amount of phosphatidylcholine increased the EE of MXD. Homogeneous dispersion, negative charge and incorporation of OAVs into the gel further improved the stability by decreasing the coalescence. There is superiority of MXD vesicular gel over MXD lotion, in its deposition in various layers of the skin, including SC, according to the skin permeation and deposition studies. There was a 10-fold increase in MXD follicular deposition for vesicular gel compared to control.

The potential application of OAVs that can self-assemble to form nanosized vesicles encapsulating MXD was shown with evidence in this study. The physiochemical attributes of MXD are improved by OAVs, by increasing follicular and skin deposition. There is considerable enhancement in MXD delivery, due to spherical morphology, desired vesicle size and better drug entrapment. Better patient compliance, efficacy and safety are seen with MXD vesicular gel for topical applications. Further in vivo studies with suitable animal models will be essential to support the efficacy seen in this study.

Key Messages
- Better patient compliance, efficacy and safety are seen with MXD vesicular gel for topical applications
- The physiochemical attributes of MXD are improved by OAVs, by increasing follicular and skin deposition
- In our experience, gel-based minoxidil (MXD) if used on tonsured scalp or trimmed scalp gives faster and better results than lotion and foam-based preparation because gel preparation has better penetration, modification of available gel preparations with incorporating OAVs would be of great benefits.

ARTICLE 46

Stability of an Extemporaneously Compounded Minoxidil Oral Suspension

Song Y, Chin ZW, Ellis D. Stability of an Extemporaneously Compounded Minoxidil Oral Suspension. Am J Health Syst Pharm. 2018;75(5):309-15.

Abstract

Purpose: To determine the stability of an extemporaneously compounded minoxidil, oral suspension under various stress and temperature conditions are reported.

Methods: Commercially available 10 mg minoxidil tablets were crushed into fine powder, and 1 mg/mL suspension was produced using predetermined amounts of two suspending vehicles, which was stored at refrigerator (4 ± 2°C) or room temperature (25 ± 2°C) in glass bottles.

Five days weekly one bottle of the suspension was removed from the refrigerated storage and was shaken, 0.5 mL of the content was discarded to simulate daily patient use. At each specified time point, using a validated high-performance liquid chromatography method, samples were analyzed in duplicate (n = 6 for each test condition). Samples pH was measured at each time point and samples were visually observed. Microbiological studies were conducted at baseline and at week 24.

Results: Throughout the 24-week study, the mean percentage of baseline minoxidil concentration remaining in all refrigerated samples exceeded 90%, with no change in redispersibility, pH, odor, microbial activity, or appearance. The suspension exhibited a color change at 4 weeks, with slight sedimentation after week 6, although minoxidil recovery exceeded 90% at week 10, during storage at room temperature.

Conclusion: A compounded, extemporaneously minoxidil oral suspension was stable when stored in refrigerator for 24 weeks. This suspension when stored at room temperature can be used for up to 3 weeks.

COMMENT

Minoxidil, a piperidino-pyrimidine derivative, is an oral vasodilator that selectively relaxes peripheral vascular smooth muscles, thus reducing blood pressure. This study aims to evaluate the chemical and physical stability and microbiological characteristics of the extemporaneously prepared minoxidil oral suspension.

In this study, tablets of minoxidil (10 mg) were crushed to a fine powder and a suspension of 1 mg/mL was produced by adding two suspending vehicles, which was stored in glass bottles at room temperature (25 ± 2°C) or in a refrigerator (4 ± 2°C). One bottle of the suspension was removed, simulating daily patient usage on weekly basis, from refrigerated storage and shaken and 0.5 mL of the contents discarded. Samples were analyzed in duplicate at specified time point using a validated high-performance liquid chromatography method.

Using buffer system consisting of Ora-Plus and Ora-Sweet SF, both of which are formulated with citric acid and sodium phosphate, a constant pH and stability of the minoxidil suspension was attained. Minoxidil suspension is demonstrated to have good stability when stored for up to 24 weeks in a refrigerator. Accelerated stability studies of minoxidil have shown that minoxidil stored at room temperature will decompose to deoxyminoxidil on exposure to heat. A significant discoloration was observed in the minoxidil suspension stored at room temperature after week 4, which might be caused by the degradation of minoxidil.

An extemporaneously compounded minoxidil oral suspension was stable for 24 weeks when stored in a refrigerator but when stored at room temperature it can be used for up to 3 weeks.

Key Messages

- The idea of oral low dose minoxidil for patterned hair loss was originated from Sinclair and group when they showed efficacy and safety of oral low dose of about 0.625 mg of minoxidil in treating female pattern hair loss (FPHL). Since this dosage formulation is not available in the market as minoxidil is available in 10 mg tablet form, compounding is necessary
- Some precautions before starting oral minoxidil:
  - Watch for side effects like low blood pressure, tachycardia and fluid retention
  - All women of child-bearing age must use effective contraception during treatment and for 1 month after stopping treatment to prevent pregnancy obtain a negative pregnancy test before start of treatment
  - Word of caution while on treatment:
    - If you notice an increase in pulse rate by more than 20 beats per minute over the normal pulse rate
    - More than 2 kg weight gain or ankle swelling
    - Shortness of breath/chest discomfort/dizziness.
- Extemporaneously compounded minoxidil oral suspension can be used for up to 3 weeks when stored at room temperature
- When stored in refrigerator, the minoxidil suspension was stable for 24 weeks.

ARTICLE 47

Efficacy of Topical Combination of 0.25% Finasteride and 3% Minoxidil Versus 3% Minoxidil Solution in Female Pattern Hair Loss: A Randomized, Double-blind, Controlled Study

Suchonwanit P, Iamsumang W, Rojhirunsakool S. Efficacy of topical combination of 0.25% finasteride and 3% minoxidil versus 3% minoxidil solution in female pattern hair loss: A randomized, double-blind, controlled study.
Am J Clin Dermatol. 2019;20(1):147-53.

Abstract

Efficacy of oral finasteride (FIN) in female pattern hair loss (FPHL) has been reported. Topical formulations of FIN have been developed in an attempt to minimize systemic adverse effects. This study compares the efficacy of combination of 3% minoxidil with 0.25% FIN to topical 3% minoxidil (MXD) in FPHL.

COMMENT

Female pattern hair loss (FPHL) is a progressive hair thinning in the crown with preservation of frontal hairline. It occurs in 6% of women aged <50 years. Topical minoxidil (MXD) 2% solution and 5% foam are the only Food and Drug Administration (FDA) approved medications. Finasteride (FIN), a selective type II 5α-reductase inhibitor, is the FDA approved treatment for male AGA but has limited its use in women due to its teratogenicity effect and also reported side effects of sexual dysfunction, depression, dizziness, increased liver enzymes and allergic reaction. To overcome its potential side effects, topical formulation has been proposed. Though efficacy of oral FIN is conflicting, Mazzarella et al. first noted the efficacy of topical FIN in FPHL in 1997.

It was a pilot, randomized, double-blind, controlled trial to evaluate the efficacy and safety of topical FIN versus topical MXD in women with FPHL. Study included 30 postmenopausal women diagnosed with FPHL, Ludwig type I, II or III. The study was conducted over 24 weeks and follow-up visits were scheduled every 8 weeks. All subjects applied study solution 1 mL, twice a day for 24 weeks, and maintained same hair style and length. Measuring hair density and diameter from baseline to week 24 using TrichoScan assessed the primary efficacy endpoint. The secondary efficacy endpoint was a global photographic assessment by investigators and subjects. To monitor the adverse events, any change in sexual function, vital signs and breast examination was routinely assessed along with estimation of serum DHT and basic laboratory parameters at baseline and 24 weeks. There were no significant statistical differences noted between the two groups but increased hair diameter was observed with FIN combination compared with MXD alone at 24 weeks after treatment. There were no adverse events in both groups except for pruritus one from each group. The baseline serum DHT levels were normal in both groups, but serum DHT levels at 24 weeks were decreased in FIN and MXD group, which indicates significant percutaneous absorption. As previous pharmacokinetic studies have demonstrated systemic absorption, this topical formulation should be used in postmenopausal women to avoid teratogenic effect and also increase risk of breast cancer due to relative estrogen excess or lack of androgens.

Key Messages

- The outcomes of topical FIN, either as monotherapy or in combination with topical MXD, were promising. It is generally well-tolerated, with only mild local adverse events reported. FIN may be considered a promising option for the treatment of FPHL as it had an additional benefit over MXD as monotherapy in terms of increasing hair diameter
- As previous pharmacokinetic studies have demonstrated systemic absorption, this topical formulation should be used in postmenopausal women to avoid teratogenic effect.

ARTICLE 48

Use of Minoxidil Sulfate versus Minoxidil Base in Androgenetic Alopecia Treatment: Friend or Foe?

Dias PC, Miot HA, Trüeb RM, et al. Use of Minoxidil Sulfate versus Minoxidil Base in Androgenetic Alopecia Treatment: Friend or Foe?
Skin Appendage Disord. 2018;4(4):349-50.

Abstract

This article aims at emphasizing the cause of treatment failures in minoxidil nonresponders, the alternate solution that is minoxidil sulfate, its practical problems with regard to low transcutaneous absorption and instability of the molecule in aqueous solution, and recommended modifications for the same.

COMMENT

Minoxidil is the FDA approved topical therapy for androgenetic alopecia. Though various mechanisms have been described for its action, the exact action is yet be defined. Minoxidil in the body gets converted into its activated metabolite minoxidil sulfate, by minoxidil sulfotransferase enzyme activity present in the outer root sheath of the hair follicle. Minoxidil sulfate is nearly 14 times more potent than plain minoxidil. However, minoxidil sulfotransferase enzyme levels vary among different individuals with some having very low levels. Such patients do not respond to the treatment. Minoxidil sulfate can be a hope in such patients. However the problem with minoxidil sulfate solution is its molecular weight of 289.3 g/mol while minoxidil has a molecular weight of 209.3 g/mol, i.e. about 40% higher. The drawback being decreased percutaneous absorption. In addition to the issue of its higher molecular weight, minoxidil sulfate is naturally unstable in aqueous solution, negatively affecting its bioavailability to the hair follicle, and increasing its irritation potential to the scalp. To overcome these issues, minoxidil sulfate would have to be used at higher concentrations (10-15%) to compensate decreased capacity of transcutaneous absorption and packaged in small volumes, because of its high degree of degradation thus avoiding scalp irritation. However large numbers of studies are required to know the efficacy and safety of this molecule.

> **Key Messages**
> - Minoxidil sulfotransferase enzyme converts minoxidil into its active form minoxidil sulfate, the lack of which results in nonresponse to minoxidil
> - Minoxidil sulfate is an alternative therapy for such patients. However the practical problems like higher molecular weight and instability of the molecule need to be addressed before recommending it as therapeutic agent
> - Recent studies show that estimation of sulfotransferase enzyme in outer root sheath is possible in biopsy specimens. If this becomes a reality in vivo, it is possible to predict response potential as well as response rate of minoxidil in patients of patterned hair loss.

ARTICLE 49

Off-label Use of Topical Minoxidil in Alopecia: A Review

Stoehr JR, Choi JN, Colavincenzo M, et al. Off-Label Use of Topical Minoxidil in Alopecia: A Review. *Am J Clin Dermatol. 2019;20(2):237-50.*

Abstract

Topical minoxidil, since after the United States Food and Drug Administration approval in 1988, has been the most utilized drug in dermatological practice for the treatment of alopecia. It's off label uses have been extended to other kinds of alopecia. There is mixed evidence for minoxidil efficacy and has been reported to be used in telogen effluvium (TE), alopecia areata (AA), scarring alopecia, eyebrow hypotrichosis, monilethrix and chemotherapy-induced alopecia (CIA).

COMMENT

This is a review article discussing off-label uses of minoxidil in alopecia. Studies, full-text articles (case reports, case series, clinical trials, and reviews), written in the English language and published from 1983 to 2017 that discussed the use of topical minoxidil in non-AGA (non-androgenetic alopecia), met the inclusion criteria for this narrative and non-systematic review.

Telogen effluvium is a type of non-inflammatory, nonscarring alopecia. It is characterized by a large amount of hair follicles entering the telogen (resting) phase and followed by shedding 3–5 months later. It may be due to an emotional or physiological stress or such as an underlying disease, surgery, pregnancy, or medication. There are limited studies showing efficacy of minoxidil in telogen effluvium (TE). A study was conducted in 2003 where mice were treated with topical minoxidil and then exposed to sonic stress, which inhibits hair growth.

The minoxidil-treated mice had reduced stress-induced hair changes, which implied a potential benefit for use of minoxidil in patients with stress-induced TE. Another study has demonstrated the efficacy of oral minoxidil (0.25–1 mg) in 36 cases of chronic TE for 1 year with significant decrease in hair shedding at 6 months and 1 year. The adverse effects were limited, and none of the patient discontinued the treatment.

Alopecia areata (AA) is a complex, immune-mediated condition characterized by clearly demarcated patches of nonscarring alopecia that are round or oval in shape and can be of severe variety with complete alopecia of the scalp in the case of alopecia totalis (AT), and complete alopecia of the entire body in alopecia universalis (AU). The mechanism of minoxidil action is by suppression of DNA synthesis and leukocyte inhibitory factor in lymphocytes, without affecting viability or migration behavior. This concluded that minoxidil topical application may be having a local immunosuppressive effect which promoted hair regrowth in AA.

In a 2014 literature review, four randomized controlled trials (RCTs) had showed some benefit of minoxidil in AA versus four RCTs showing no significant effect. In 1980, two trials were conducted which used 1% minoxidil either applied once or twice daily. Both studies demonstrated that there was cosmetically acceptable hair regrowth in minoxidil treated group. The authors did not observe topical or systemic side effects. But response in severe cases of AT and AU was minimal. In another two studies, authors proposed that minoxidil may be effective in maintaining prednisolone-induced hair growth in AA patients.

Another double-blind, crossover study comprising of 15 subjects from 1985 had used 3% minoxidil solution on subjects with AT. There was vellus or intermediate hair growth in eight subjects but was not therapeutically significant. There are many other studies which demonstrated that there was no cosmetically acceptable hair regrowth (CAHR) in patients with severe forms of AA when treated with minoxidil. This concludes that as the severity of the AA increases, the efficacy of minoxidil for its treatment may decline.

In pediatric AA, the advantages of minoxidil in treatment are not clear and children may be at more risk of adverse effects from the drug. Five such cases reported either no benefit or cosmetically inappropriate hypertrichosis as side effect. One of the report showed that three adolescents (aged 10–14 years) had cardiovascular effects, including palpitations, dizziness and sinus tachycardia, after using topical minoxidil for AA for 1 month, which resolved with elimination of drug.

Frontal fibrosing alopecia (FFA) is identified as a clinical variant of lichen planopilaris. A retrospective review of 355 patients, one of the largest review, reported that 78% of patients (n = 276) used topical minoxidil and corticosteroids as part of their therapy, with variable efficacy. There have been no controlled trials, minoxidil use in FFA has only been described anecdotally as an adjuvant therapy. In 15 case reports series comparing amongst various FFA treatment modalities, authors found three studies (n = 5) where minoxidil was used in treating FFA. Their result was categorized for efficacy; three patients showed "no effect" and two patients showed "partial effect".

Central centrifugal cicatricial alopecia (CCCA) is having unknown etiology and affects African American women, characterized by progressive alopecia beginning at the vertex of the scalp with follicular degeneration, fibrosis and inflammation. Some authors report the use of minoxidil in combination with other treatments. Two studies, one retrospective review and one case report, suggests that minoxidil is not helpful in treating CCCA.

Traction alopecia (TA) occurs due to tension on the hair inflicted by certain hair styles. The early stages of TA are nonscarring and reversible, that is why there is potential benefit of minoxidil in patients who have had the condition for a short time. A case report of two patients had shown significant hair regrowth on visual assessment using 2% minoxidil alone in patients who had been longstanding TA (over 1 year) after the traumatic hairstyles had ceased.

Eyebrow hypotrichosis, a cosmetic concern, can be because of various etiologies. It can be idiopathic, due to trauma, medical, or surgical treatment, or may be associated with systemic diseases such as hypothyroidism, or can occur due to another alopecic disease such as AA or FFA. A split face study comparing efficacy of 2% minoxidil with placebo in 39 patients has found that after 16 weeks topical minoxidil was well tolerated and effective. In another split face study, a comparison between topical minoxidil and bimatoprost was done which involved 27 subjects. The outcomes were compared for global assessment, hair diameter measurement, and patient satisfaction. The results after 16 weeks revealed that both treatments were equally efficacious in improving eyebrow hair diameter and patient satisfaction.

Monilethrix, a rare genodermatosis, which manifests clinically as brittle, fragile hair with beading of the hair shaft, and keratosis pilaris has been treated with minoxidil. A case series of four patients conducted in 2011 on patients in age ranging from 5 years to 47 years, who were treated with topical minoxidil for 1 year with evaluations done at 6 and 12 months. The authors found out an increase of normal hair shaft via videodermatoscopy and noted no adverse effects.

Chemotherapy-induced alopecia (CIA) is caused due to apoptotic damage to proliferating hair follicle cells, resulting in either telogen or anagen effluvium. Scalp cooling is the most promising treatment for the prevention of CIA. In treatment of CIA, minoxidil has been examined in various studies and reviews for prevention and treatment. In a double-blind study comprising of 48 patients with various types of solid tumors, patients were randomly divided into control and placebo groups. Each group was given either minoxidil or placebo to apply twice daily starting 24 hour before their first chemotherapy treatment. After two cycles of doxorubicin, the severity and extent of alopecia was evaluated. Almost 90% of the treatment group and 91% of the placebo group patients had severe hair loss requiring the use of a wig. The authors concluded treatment had no preventive effect. Although minoxidil may not be preventive, it was found to be efficacious for the treatment of CIA in a randomized, double-blind trial. That study comprised of 20 women; the period of baldness was reduced by mean 50.2 days, in patients treated with minoxidil. The patients did not report scalp hair loss even after discontinuation of minoxidil use.

Another variant of CIA is permanent CIA (PCIA) which is characterized by alopecia that persists for 6 or more months after stopping chemotherapy. Topical minoxidil is ineffective once PCIA has been established. A study involving 14 subjects showed that there was no benefit in hair regrowth after 3+ months of using the topical minoxidil (2 or 5%). A single case report showed subjective hair regrowth at 6 weeks of treatment in a patient who had PCIA for 16 months after chemotherapy and bone marrow transplant with oral minoxidil (1 mg daily). It also showed histological change like decreased telogen follicles, reversed miniaturization at 2 years of treatment, with no side effects.

> **Key Messages**
> - In spite of lack of conclusive evidence, minoxidil is still used in treatment of AA and scarring alopecia
> - Minoxidil has a role in the treatment of eyebrow hypotrichosis, monilethrix and early TA, as well as for reducing the duration of CIA as demonstrated with various studies.

ARTICLE 50

A Comment on the Post-Finasteride Syndrome

Rezende HD, Reis Dias MFRG, Trueb RM. A Comment on the Post-Finasteride Syndrome. *Int J Trichol. 2018;10(6):255-61.*

Abstract

The Post-Finasteride Syndrome (PFS) has been claimed by some of the nondermatologists, neuroendocrinological research, case reports, and uncontrolled studies in men who have taken oral finasteride for hair loss or benign prostatic hyperplasia. The incidence of persistent sexual, mental and physical side effects is still unknown. The scrutiny of these studies done by hair experts showed strong bias in case selection and a significant nocebo effect. The best way to alleviate the emotional distress related to hair loss is to effectively treat the condition causing the problem.

COMMENT

It is the aim of this commentary to provide information on, how to react in case of drug-related adverse events, issues of fertility and malignancy, and management of the post-Finasteride syndrome (PFS). Finasteride is a major breakthrough in the treatment of male pattern hair loss. In 2012, Sato and Takeda reported on efficacy and safety of 1 mg oral finasteride for treatment of male pattern hair loss in the so far largest population study of enrolled 3,177 Japanese men. Adverse reactions occurred only in 0.7% of men. Dutasteride has been proposed for enhancement of efficacy in the treatment of male pattern hair loss due to its dual 5α-reductase inhibition.

Post-Finasteride syndrome has been claimed to occur in men who have taken oral finasteride to treat either hair loss or benign prostatic hyperplasia. Reported symptoms include loss of libido, erectile dysfunction, reduction in penis size, penile curvature or reduced sensation, gynecomastia, muscle atrophy, cognitive impairment, severely dry skin, and depression which were claimed to continue despite quitting finasteride. This has led to a lot of sufferings with reduced quality of life.

The Post-Finasteride Syndrome Foundation (www.pfsfoundation.org) is a nonprofit organization dedicated to fund research on understanding biologic mechanisms and treatments of the PFS while improving public awareness of the condition.

There are scientific studies in rodents that showed finasteride may reduce the concentration of several neuroactive steroids important for neurogenesis and neuronal survival. An important neurosteroid is allopregnanolone (ALLO), a metabolite of dihydroprogesterone. ALLO is a potent ligand of the inhibitory GABA-barbiturate receptor. Less ALLO, as a consequence of finasteride treatment, could alter GABAergic transmission. Since neurosteroids are believed to have anxiolytic, antidepressant and memory enhancement properties and play a role in neuroprotection, the decrease of neurosteroid biosynthesis through inhibition of the enzyme 5α-reductase required to synthesize these neurosteroids, may contribute to the respective psychiatric adverse events.

Post-Finasteride syndrome represents a nocebo reaction or a real drug adverse effect that is irrelevant, but the best way to alleviate the emotional distress is to treat the problem. The basis for this assumption of finasteride adverse events would be assessed by sexual hormones, sexual orientation, handedness and cognition might all be interrelated, presumably due to overall lateralized processes of the brain. A study on the relationship of the digit (or 2D: 4D) ratio to the frequency of finasteride-related mental and sexual adverse effects has been proposed.

It is important to take history of depression or sexual dysfunction before starting treatment, since pre-existing mental health disorders among finasteride users may put this subset of patients at an increased risk of developing emotional disorders related to finasteride therapy. It is important to educate patient rather than a simple transfer of information. Understanding, emotion, satisfaction, rapport and empathy are among the factors involved. This maximizes patient benefit and safety. Patients frequently become preoccupied with side effects when they are reluctant to undergo treatment, and some physicians also overestimate side effects. Nocebo effect has been revealed in patients who were informed of potential sexual adverse effects versus patients who were not informed.

In any case of adverse effects, oral finasteride should be stopped. Since the plasma half lifetime of dutasteride (3–5 weeks) is significantly longer than that of finasteride (from 5 hours to 8 hours), it is advisable to start patients on oral finasteride initially and then switch on to dutasteride if there is no satisfactory result at 6 months. Switch from oral finasteride to topical minoxidil may be considered in anticipation of age-related more frequent sexual function-related problems. As there is no evidence of androgen deficiency, persistent steroid 5α-reductase inhibition or androgen insensitivity, finasteride users are unlikely to benefit from treatment with testosterone or any other androgen.

> **Key Messages**
> - In the management of the PFS, attention must be focused on the treatment of depression and sexual symptoms
> - Preventive measures include refraining from prescribing oral finasteride to patients with a personal history of depression, sexual dysfunction or fertility problems
> - In case of adverse effects, stopping oral finasteride treatment and adding topical finasteride is best alternative with good efficacy which was showed in few randomized controlled trials and prospective studies.

ARTICLE 51

Low Dose Daily Aspirin Reduces Topical Minoxidil Efficacy in Androgenetic Alopecia Patients

Goren A, Sharma A, Dhurat R, et al. Low dose daily aspirin reduces topical minoxidil efficacy in androgenetic alopecia patients.
Dermatol Ther. 2018;31(6):e12741.

Abstract

The article describes a cohort study to report the effect of low-dose daily aspirin use on the efficacy of topical minoxidil. A cohort of 24 subjects were included, 50% were initially predicted to be responders to minoxidil. Follicular sulfotransferase enzymatic activity was estimated following 14 days of oral aspirin administration. However, only 27% of the subjects were predicted to respond to topical minoxidil after 14 days of study period compared to initial prediction of 50%. Thus oral aspirin inhibits sulfotransferase activity in hair follicles also, thereby affecting minoxidil response in androgenetic alopecia (AGA).

COMMENT

Minoxidil is the mainstay therapy for androgenetic alopecia (AGA), the only preparation USFDA approved as an OTC drug for the treatment of AGA. Minoxidil is converted to its active form, minoxidil sulfate, by the action of sulfotransferase enzymes present in the outer root sheath (ORS) of hair follicles. Thus, its efficacy is limited by the enzyme activity in ORS of hair. Salicylic acid and aspirin (a derivative of salicylic acid) are significant inhibitors of human liver sulfotransferases. The authors have made an attempt to study the effect of low-dose daily aspirin administration on the sulfotransferase enzyme activity in the ORS of hair follicles utilizing the minoxidil response assay.

A cohort of 24 male subjects with AGA was recruited, subjects were provided 14 tablets of 75 mg aspirin, one tablet per day, and plucked hair samples were collected during the visit on the 14th day and sent to analysis. Twenty two patients returned after 14 days. Twelve (55%) subjects showed significant reduction ($p < 0.0001$) in follicular sulfotransferase enzymatic activity, following 14 days of aspirin therapy. Minoxidil response test (MRT) initially had predicted that 11 (50%) of the 22 subjects may respond to topical minoxidil; following 14 days of aspirin administration, only 6 (27%) subjects were predicted to respond to topical minoxidil.

In conclusion, low-dose oral aspirin, being a commonly prescribed drug worldwide in cardiovascular states especially coronary heart disease, and its inhibitory activity of sulfotransferase enzymes in the human hair ORS, reduces the efficacy of minoxidil; therefore, chronic use of low-dose aspirin would also interfere with the efficacy of topical minoxidil treatment in AGA.

The demographic profile of AGA patients, shows that the disease activity and severity is considerably affecting the population which is 20–40 years of age. The same group is also showing increased morbidity due to cardiovascular diseases and neurological diseases where aspirin has to be given for an indefinite period. Clinicians have to remember that minoxidil treatment of AGA is a relative contraindication in cardiovascular patients, added to this, the observation made in this study points toward reduced efficacy of minoxidil. In background of this, prescribing minoxidil in patients who are on the aspirin has to be critical and judgmental. Instead nonminoxidil options appear to be safer and better.

Key Message

- Patient's aspirin regimen needs to be considered prior to initiating minoxidil therapy for AGA as it can affect outcomes.

ARTICLE 52

A Randomized, Double-blind Controlled Study of the Efficacy and Safety of Topical Solution of 0.25% Finasteride Admixed with 3% Minoxidil versus 3% Minoxidil Solution in the Treatment of Male Androgenetic Alopecia

Suchonwanit P, Srisuwanwattana P, Chalermroj N, et al. A randomized, double-blind controlled study of the efficacy and safety of topical solution of 0.25% finasteride admixed with 3% minoxidil vs. 3% minoxidil solution in the treatment of male androgenetic alopecia.
J Eur Acad Dermatol Venereol. 2018;32(12):2257-63.

Abstract

This study compares the efficacy and safety of topical 0.25% finasteride + 3% minoxidil (MX) versus 3% MX solution alone in 40 male androgenetic alopecia (AGA) patients for 24 weeks. The combination therapy was superior to 3% MX solution alone for promoting hair.

COMMENT

Androgenetic alopecia (AGA) is characterized by a progressive miniaturization of terminal scalp hair with dihydrotestosterone (DHT) being the important causative factor. Finasteride, 5α-reductase inhibitor, 1 mg daily and topical minoxidil (MX) 5% are the only two FDA-approved drugs for managing androgenetic alopecia (AGA). To minimize systemic adverse effects, particularly sexual dysfunction, topical finasteride 0.005–0.5% has been suspected to be a potential alternative option. The recent studies have shown the ability of topical 0.25% finasteride to reduce plasma and scalp DHT levels. This was equivalent to oral finasteride 1 mg daily while the plasma exposure was about 9-fold lower.

This was a randomized double-blind study aimed to determine the clinical efficacy and safety of a topical formulation of 0.25% finasteride admixed with 3% minoxidil (FMX), in comparison with 3% MX solution in the treatment of male AGA for 24 weeks. All subjects maintained the same hair color, style and length. The primary efficacy endpoint was the change from baseline, in hair density and hair diameter within a 1-cm diameter on the vertex at week 8, 16 and 24 assessed by trichoscopy, photographing with a Folliscope®. The global photographic assessment was by both investigators and patients.

The FMX was significantly superior to MX in increasing hair density at week 16 and

24, as well as in increasing hair diameter at week 24. FMX showed significant superiority over MX in promoting hair growth at week 24. There were neither serious adverse events nor sexual problems reported in both groups except for flaky scalp and scalp pruritus in few patients. Pregnant and childbearing women must not use finasteride solutions (genital defects in the male fetus) and also it is not clear how much systemic absorption takes place when finasteride is applied topically. The limitations of this study were no long-term follow-up data, and no evaluation of scalp DHT levels was done.

Key Messages

- A 0.25% finasteride solution is equivalent to that of finasteride 1 mg in reducing plasma and scalp DHT levels
- The FMX solution yielded a better therapeutic efficacy over 3% MX solution in treating male AGA
- One of the important endpoint of this study was assessment of plasma DHT which is 9-fold lower than oral, however scalp DHT levels were not assessed which is the limitation of this study
- Finasteride solution has high resistance to biodegradation hence it must not be thrown in the trash/drain or flushed down in the toilet as it can accumulate in adipose tissue of aquatic organisms.

ARTICLE 53

The Post-Finasteride Syndrome: Clinical Manifestation of Drug-induced Epigenetics due to Endocrine Disruption

Traish AM. The Post-finasteride syndrome: Clinical manifestation of drug-induced epigenetics due to endocrine disruption.
Curr Sex Health Rep. 2018;10(3):88-103.

Abstract

The article is a review on Post-Finasteride syndrome (PFS). The adverse effects of finasteride are well-known, the symptom cluster are often dismissed. Additionally, there is lack of comprehensive understanding of the biochemical and pathophysiological mechanisms causing PFS. The article attempts to throw light on physiology, pathophysiology and clinical management of patients with PFS.

COMMENT

In this review, physiology of neurosteroids in relation to Post-Finasteride syndrome (PFS) is elaborated. A 5α-reductase(5α-R) reaction is the rate-limiting step in the synthesis of 3α,5α steroid derivatives. Neuroactive steroids such as 3α,5α-androstane, 17β-diol (3α-diol), 3α,5α-tetrahydroprogesterone (3α,5αTHP;), 3α,5α tetrahydrodeoxycorticosterone (3α,5α-THDOC), 3β,5α-androstane, 17β-diol (3β-diol), and isopregnanolone regulate specific functions in peripheral and central nervous system, not directly related to steroid levels in the blood. Several neurosteroids act by auto- or paracrine mechanisms involving both regulation of target gene expression and effects on membrane receptors (including neurotransmitters).

Post-Finasteride syndrome encompasses sexual dysfunction (SD), erectile dysfunction (ED), loss of libido, depression, suicidal ideation, anxiety, panic attacks, insomnia and cognitive dysfunction. Finasteride treatment impairs biosynthesis and action of neurosteroids, and modulates gamma amino butyric acid receptors causing a host of physiological functions, ranging from sexual activity, mood and cognition.

Finasteride-induced epigenetic changes in gene expression, including upregulation of androgen receptors (AR), increased histone acetylation, and methylation results in impairment of dopaminergic signaling manifested in anxiety, depression and suicidal ideation. Two polymorphisms in *AR* gene, namely CAG (rs4045402) and GGN (rs3138869), have a role in finasteride sensitivity; authors proposed that polymorphisms are frequent among patients with androgenetic alopecia (AGA) and PFS. Modulation of tissue AR levels is implicated in long-term side effects of finasteride use. Finasteride acts as an endocrine disruptor of neurosteroid biosynthesis and activity; elicits undesirable epigenetic changes and persistent symptoms even after drug discontinuation.

The adverse sexual effects in PFS leads to decreased self-esteem, quality of life and ability to maintain an intimate relationship. The SD side effects of 5α-R inhibitors may be long-lasting and persistent. Ali et al. found that persistent SD is a potential risk of low-dose finasteride for AGA therapy in young men, and this risk contributes to SI. Chiriaco et al. found in their study that adverse side effects persisted for over 6 months after finasteride discontinuation. Guo et al. also found in their study that the median time of persistent SD after discontinuation was 339 days, primary and secondary analysis of persistent SD were 2.19 (crude) and 1.62 (adjusted) for finasteride compared to 1 in the omeprazole group and 2.41 and 2.73, respectively, suggesting an increased risk of persistent SD with finasteride.

There are limitations of studies assessing adverse effects of 5α-reductase Inhibitors as there are inadequate data reporting and poor assessment utilizing non-validated questionnaires to address the scope and magnitude of the adverse side effects. From patient perspective, patients have reported fatigue, social isolation, cognitive dysfunction (brain fog) and insomnia causing suicidal attempts and even suicide. From clinician perspective, it should be pointed out that men taking finasteride for treatment should be counseled well prior to prescription.

> **Key Message**
>
> - Finasteride inhibition of 5α-reductases results in reduced biosynthesis and metabolism of neurosteroids causing attenuating or silencing of signaling by androgen receptors and neurotransmitter receptors and therefore manifests in as PFS.

ARTICLE 54

A Randomized Study of Biomimetic Peptides Efficacy and Impact on the Growth Factors Expression in the Hair Follicles of Patients with Telogen Effluvium

Kubanov AA, Gallyamova YA, Korableva OA. A randomized study of biomimetic peptides efficacy and impact on the growth factors expression in the hair follicles of patients with telogen effluvium.
J App Pharm Sci. 2018;8(04):015-022.

Abstract

Biomimetic peptides consist of amino acid residues and are used to treat hair loss. This is a randomized study to know the expression of growth factors [vascular endothelial growth factor (VEGF), keratinocyte growth factor (KGF), epidermal growth factor (EGF), transforming growth factor beta 1 (TGF-β1)] in the hair follicle of patients with telogen effluvium and healthy individuals and to evaluate the efficacy of biomimetic peptides in telogen effluvium. A total of 30 female patients with telogen effluvium were randomized to two groups, group I treated with biomimetic peptides and group II were placebo. A punch biopsy was taken from the frontotemporal areas before and after the therapy, and subjected to immunofluorescence study. Trichoscopy and phototrichography was done to know the therapeutic efficacy of biomimetic peptides in telogen effluvium. There was change in the expression of VEGF, KGF and TGF-β1 growth factors in telogen effluvium as opposed to the healthy ones. Upon completion of treatment, a significant increase in the VEGF and EGF expression, and a decrease in KGF and TGF-β1 expression were noted. This study proved the effectiveness of biomimetic peptides for women with telogen effluvium.

COMMENT

The role of regulatory substances in hair cycling is highlighted by the fundamental biochemical and cytogenetic research. These include intracellular signaling pathways, transcription factors, growth factor families and receptors, cytokines and neurotrophins.

The polypeptide growth factors that are referred to as trophic regulatory substances are given special considerations. A variety of effects are exerted by these factors on various cells: inhibit or stimulate cell proliferation chemotaxis, and differentiation. Recently the growth factors which are regulators of the hair growth cycle are established. Growth factors can induce cell proliferation of dermal fibroblasts and vascular endothelium, delaying catagen and prolonging anagen onset in a hair follicle. VEGF is very important in the development of hair. It promotes growth, determines the structure, differentiation, and duration of the hair shaft and hair follicle in vivo.

In this well-designed novel study, the effect of biomimetic peptides on growth factor expression in a hair follicle and therapeutic efficacy in female patients with telogen effluvium was assessed. A lotion based on biomimetic peptides (2 mL) was topically applied on the scalp of group I patients and followed by microneedle therapy (needle size of 0.2 mm). Treatment with normal saline (NS) followed by microneedle therapy was followed in patients of group II. The analysis of the phototrichogram and trichoscopy indices in the occipital and parietal regions (the number of follicular units per square centimeter, hair density, the percentage of hair in the anagen stage, the hair diameter) before treatment, after treatment, and at follow-up of month 2 and 6 showed a statistically significant higher increase in hair percentage in the anagen stage in females of the main group, as compared to control group. The percentage of the telogen and the anagen hair reached normal values, in patients treated with biomimetic peptides. Perifollicular vascularization can be improved by use of biomimetic peptide treatment, which leads to intensified hair growth by improved blood flow. TGF-β is a powerful growth inhibitor of various cell types, including epithelial cells; following biomimetic peptide treatment, a reduction in TGF-β expression indicates reduced apoptosis in patients after treatment, in comparison to the sample before treatment.

With this literature, authors showed that topical application of biomimetic peptides are safe, followed by microneedle therapy. It is to be noted that wounding itself brings about the changes in metabolic process of hair follicle regeneration and development, but in this study upregulation and downregulation of growth factors was compared with NS as placebo proving the efficacy of biomimetic peptides. The use of microneedling is to ensure and enhance penetration of these peptides as transcutaneous absorption of these molecules is hindered by their molecular size. Subjectively, patients well tolerated the treatment, with no noticeable side effects, and no patients from the observation group were excluded. Withdrawal syndrome was not observed at the end of treatment. Phototrichographic parameters were analyzed by the authors and they concluded, patients with telogen effluvium, experience reduced hair thinning due to anagen stimulation and telogen shortening due to anagen prolongation. Anagen initiation is evidenced objectively by the presence of juvenile hair and anagen prolongation is indicated by increased number of units over the treatment period.

Key Messages

- Growth factors can induce cell proliferation of dermal fibroblasts and vascular endothelium, delaying catagen and prolonging anagen onset in a hair follicle
- Perifollicular vascularization can be improved by use of biomimetic peptide treatment, which leads to intensified hair growth by improved blood flow
- Following biomimetic peptide treatment, a reduction in TGF-β expression indicates reduced apoptosis in patients after treatment, in comparison to the sample before treatment
- This study brings some evidence for biomimetic peptide therapy in chronic telogen effluvium questionable efficacy.

ARTICLE 55

Study of Vasodilating and Regenerative Effect of the Gel with Nettle Juice intended for Telogen Effluvium Treatment

Ivanivna FM, Petrivna PN, Mykolaivna FS, et al. Study of vasodilating and regenerative effect of the gel with nettle juice intended for telogen effluvium treatment.
J Appl Pharm Sci. 2018;8(01):093-7.

Abstract

Hair loss in women is a major cause of psychological distress. Among the various reasons, telogen effluvium (TE) remains one of the common causes of hair loss. This study was conducted to see the vasodilating and regenerative effects of nettle juice in the management of TE. The effects of topical application of the gel in wool growth in rats were studied. The authors concluded that application of nettle juice accelerated the wool growth rate in rats.

COMMENT

Telogen effluvium (TE) is the most common cause of diffuse hair loss in women of reproductive age. It is usually multifactorial. A lot of plant-derived products are used in the management of TE. Stinging nettle leaves and stems contain a wide range of biologically active substances like organic (formic, pantothenic) and hydroxycinnamic (chlorogenic, caffeic, ferulic) acid, flavonoids (routine, quercetin, campherol), chlorophyll, organically bound silicon, a complex of vitamins. These substances are known to enhance blood circulation and exhibit regenerative properties of hair follicle cells. Due to these properties, infusions, masks, and juices are used to manage TE. The authors developed a cosmetic gel with nettle juice and the study was carried out to test the effects of that gel on hair growth of rats.

According to this study, developed gel stimulated the recovery of damaged hair follicle growth, increased the thickness of the hair, reduced the number of dystrophic hair and caused significant dilation of blood vessels in the reticular dermis. The hair follicle density also increased which may be due to stimulated hair follicle genesis.

Nettle leaf seeds and flowers are known to have a lot of medical benefits, primarily these compounds have irritant property notably causing vasodilatation by mast cell degranulation. As these results can be extrapolated to hair disorders, it might suit best for alopecia areata.

Key Message

- The developed gel with nettle juice appears to be a promising treatment option for TE.

ARTICLE 56

Comparative Evaluation between Two Nutritional Supplements in the Improvement of Telogen Effluvium

Addor FA, Donato LC, Melo CS. Comparative evaluation between two nutritional supplements in the improvement of telogen effluvium.
Clin Cosmet Investig Dermatol. 2018;11:431.

Abstract

Telogen effluvium (TE) is the most common cause of diffuse hair loss in women of reproductive age. Dietary supplements are commonly prescribed in the management of TE. In this study, the authors have compared two types of nutritional supplements as monotherapy over a period of 6 months. Group 1: a supplement composed of zinc, biotin, iron, vitamins A, C, E and B complex, folic acid, magnesium, and amino acids of keratin and collagen; group 2: calcium pantothenate cystine, thiamine nitrate, medicinal yeast, keratin and aminobenzoic acid. Clinical evaluation at 180 days showed significant improvement in group 1.

COMMENT

In telogen effluvium (TE), there is a shortening of the anagen phase and precipitation of the telogen phase, resulting in loss of total loss of hair volume. TE causes significant morbidity in women. The causes of TE are multifactorial, nutritional deficiency being the one most described. Nutritional supplements are indicated in TE due to deficiencies like weight loss, dietary disorders and malabsorption. As the cells in the hair follicles are rapidly dividing with high metabolic rate next to bone marrow, they are very sensitive to any nutritional deprivation. Other causes of TE-like childbirth or systemic diseases may also be associated with nutrient defects. In this study, two combinations of nutrition supplements were provided to females with idiopathic TE, to study their effects with respect to improvement in signs and symptoms. Patients were randomized into two groups—group 1: Total 60 participants used the product composed of zinc, biotin, iron, vitamins A, C, E and B complex, folic acid, magnesium, and amino acids of keratin and collagen; group 2: Total 60 participants used the product, composed of calcium pantothenate cystine, thiamine nitrate, medicinal yeast, keratin and aminobenzoic acid. Supplementation of biotin in high doses or more than 5 mg/day could be detrimental to hair growth and high biotin supplementation can result in excessive shedding.

The group 1 showed statistically significant results for the clinical parameters of hair quality, hair shine and hair strength as compared to group 2. This study points toward that, in idiopathic TE, micronutrient deficiencies should be suspected. Even borderline nutritional deficiencies which may not be reflected in the laboratory estimations can precipitate TE. Zinc is involved in the synthesis of proteins and nucleic acids, having an important role in various metabolic pathways and cellular functions. B-complex vitamins, in particular, biotin and folic acid, play a decisive role in the hair cycle. The possible benefit of the use of antioxidants in TE is supported by the associated etiological factors, especially when there are associated systemic inflammatory processes.

Key Message

◉ *Telogen effluvium is the most common cause for diffuse hair loss in women, and nutritional supplements should be provided irrespective of the etiology, as TE is often multifactorial.*

ARTICLE 57

Efficacy and Safety of a Topical Botanical in Female Androgenetic Alopecia: A Randomized, Single-blinded, Vehicle-controlled Study

Katoulis AC, Liakou AI, Alevizou A, et al. Efficacy and safety of a topical botanical in female androgenetic alopecia: a randomized, single-blinded, vehicle-controlled study.
Skin Appendage Disord. 2018;4:160-5.

Abstract

Background: Androgenetic alopecia (AGA) is a difficult-to-treat skin disorder, especially in females. A novel topical botanical lotion has been approved for its management. It acts by increasing perifollicular Langerhans and mast cells, Bcl-2 and perifollicular collagen.
We aimed to evaluate the safety and efficacy of this lotion in females.

Methods: Forty women with AGA were randomized to apply the placebo or active lotion, twice a day for 24 weeks. Subjects were evaluated by clinical examination, photographic documentation, trichogram (anagen to telogen ratio), and quality of life evaluation (DLQI) at 0, 12 and 24 weeks.

Results: The clinical evaluation demonstrated a higher hair density in the intervention group (stable in 3.8%, moderate in 88.5%, and great improvement in 7.7%). DLQI improved from 4 to 3 in the intervention group (p <0.001) and the self-assessment score increased from 4.5 to 6.0 (24 weeks). The mean anagen to telogen ratio in the control group was 2.2, 3.8, and 3.3 at 0, 12, and 24 weeks, respectively, whereas in the intervention group it was 2.1, 3.9, and 6.0 at 0, 12, and 24 weeks, respectively.

Conclusion: Remarkable efficacy and improvement of quality of life of patients with high degree of patient satisfaction was seen with the use of new topical botanical lotion.

COMMENT

Androgenetic alopecia (AGA) or pattern hair loss is a progressive noncicatricial alopecia characterized by miniaturization in which there is a gradual conversion of thick, pigmented terminal hair into vellus hair. Although much progress has been made in the treatment of AGA, especially among females, it still remains a great challenge. A novel formula (CG210®) based on seed, onion, lemon, and cocoa extracts has been approved as a treatment option for AGA. The aim of the authors was to evaluate the safety and efficacy of this botanical lotion in female pattern baldness.

This randomized, single-blinded, vehicle-controlled study was conducted for duration of 12 months, consisting of 40 women, clinically diagnosed with AGA. The study population was assigned to apply either the active lotion or the vehicle, twice daily, for 24 weeks. A standardized photographic documentation, DLQI, and trichogram were done. At each visit, the participants were asked to grade their level of satisfaction with the treatment.

Results showed an increased hair density in the majority of patients receiving the active lotion, the change in quality of life was in favor of the active treatment. The anagen to telogen ratio also significantly increased following active lotion application. The lotion used in this study increased Bcl-2 expression, an anti-apoptotic protein that prolongs the anagen phase and cell survival. It prevents follicular miniaturization and fibrosis by downregulating inflammation by increasing the number of mast cells and Langerhans cells in the perifollicular area. The efficacy of this botanical preparation is validated when the anagen to telogen ratio is restored to normal. CG210 seems to be a novel, promising treatment of female AGA.

The new topical botanical lotion has showed remarkable efficacy, with a high degree of patient satisfaction and improvement of their quality of life. The need for comparison with minoxidil may support its use as a first-line choice in the treatment of AGA.

Key Messages
- The anagen to telogen ratio is considered to be a valid indicator of the follicle activity and its restoration to normal appears to be a strong documentation of the efficacy of this new botanical
- Almost all patients clinically improved after receiving the active lotion over a 24-week period
- Lot of molecules as peptides and natural extracts from plants are making news in treating hair loss of different etiologies. Well-designed case-control studies need to be done to prove their efficacy.

ARTICLE 58

Tofacitinib for the Treatment of Alopecia Areata in Preadolescent Children

Craiglow BG, King BA. Tofacitinib for the treatment of alopecia areata in preadolescent children. *J Am Acad Dermatol. 2019;80(2):568-570.*

Abstract
Alopecia areata (AA) is a commonly encountered cause of hair loss in children. It has severe phenotypic forms which can significantly affect the quality of life. Janus kinase (JAK) inhibitors are showing promising results and hence are being tried in AA and trials have reported promising results.

COMMENT

Alopecia areata (AA) is one of the most common cause of focal atrichia in childhood with limited treatment options; paving way as well as demanding newer research options in therapeutics for optimal results. Janus kinase (JAK) inhibitors are emerging as a promising treatment targeting at the molecular level in the etiopathogenesis of AA.

The safety profile of tofacitinib in the pediatric population is not yet well established. Though the use of tofacitinib in few case series has been reported, it's use in preadolescent group, the age most vulnerable for AA and treatment response is lacking.

The authors have presented a therapeutic research paper (case series) on the efficacy of oral tofacitinib in four pediatric patients aged 8-10 years who had failed to conventional treatments. Three patients were initiated oral tofacitinib 5 mg twice daily, fourth started on 5 mg once daily for 3 months, with no regrowth dose escalated to twice daily. This case series has included only preadolescent group, severity wise the initial Severity of Alopecia Tool (SALT) scoring was 100 in all four patients, alopecia universalis was present in three of them; other had alopecia totalis, thus severe patterns were considered for systemic tofacitinib therapy. Counseling and risks were explained, complete hemogram, metabolic and lipid profile were performed [baseline and periodic (after 1 month, every 3-4 months thereafter)].

Complete regrowth was appreciated by two patients (by 3 months in one patient, 6 months in another) and a satisfactory response of 62% regrowth in one patient. Patient whose dose escalation was done after 3 months of single dosage, showed scanty regrowth even after taking twice daily. More than 50% regrowth of eyebrows in two patients was also noted.

The article succeeds in providing evidence of optimal regrowth following the use of tofacitinib for alopecia universalis and alopecia totalis in preadolescent children, yet small sample size, unknown safety profile and long-term efficacy warrant further research and need for well-designed prospective trials.

Key Messages

- Oral tofacitinib, a JAK inhibitor can be considered in severe alopecia areata, recalcitrant to conventional therapies with psychosocial impairment even in pediatric population provided immunodeficiency states are ruled out
- Counseling, parenteral consent, baseline and periodic complete hemogram, metabolic and lipid profile and zoster vaccination are mandatory.

ARTICLE 59

Tofacitinib for the Treatment of Lichen Planopilaris: A Case Series

Yang CC, Khanna T, Sallee B, et al. Tofacitinib for the treatment of lichen planopilaris: A case series. *Dermatol Ther. 2018;31(6):e12656.*

Abstract

Tofacitinib, a Janus kinase (JAK) inhibitor, has been effective in treating alopecia areata where upregulation of interferon and JAK signaling may play a role. This is a retrospective study of

10 patients with recalcitrant lichen planopilaris (LPP) treated with oral tofacitinib. Patients received oral tofacitinib, 5 mg twice or three times daily for 2–19 months as either alone or adjunctive therapy like intralesional triamcinolone, hydroxychloroquine and topical tacrolimus. Treatment with oral tofacitinib either as monotherapy or adjunctive therapy had measurable improvement in recalcitrant LPP.

COMMENT

Lichen planopilaris (LPP) is a primary lymphocytic cicatricial alopecia of unclear etiology and treatment is often unsuccessful. This was a retrospective study of 10 patients with LPP who were treated with pan-Janus kinase (JAK) inhibitor, oral tofacitinib. JAK inhibition may reduce interferon (IFN)-mediated inflammation associated with LPP and prevent further hair follicle destruction.

Lichen Planopilaris Activity Index (LPPAI) is a scoring index that records patient's symptoms (pruritus, pain, burning), a measure of activity (the anagen pull test), signs (erythema, perifollicular erythema and scale) and extension of disease. All essential laboratory blood investigations were monitored during the therapy.

Dose of tofacitinib 5 mg twice a day with the duration ranging from 2 months to 19 months was given for eight patients and used as monotherapy in five patients. Adjunctive therapies were used in five patients, which included intralesional triamcinolone (two patients), intralesional triamcinolone and hydroxychloroquine (one patient), hydroxychloroquine (one patient) and intralesional triamcinolone with tacrolimus ointment (one patient).

The LPPAI scores showed significant improvement post-treatment. No significant adverse events were noted except weight gain in one patient and the treatment had to be discontinued. Limiting factors in this study are small sample size and retrospective and heterogeneous patient group. Improvements were seen in patients using tofacitinib monotherapy and with other concomitant treatment suggesting that tofacitinib may be a promising strategy for treating LPP which requires multiple approach.

Key Messages

- Lichen planopilaris is a primary lymphocytic cicatricial alopecia of unclear etiology
- The JAK inhibition may reduce IFN-mediated inflammation associated with LPP and prevent further hair follicle destruction
- The JAK inhibition with oral tofacitinib, 5 mg twice a day, may be a promising strategy for treating LPP
- This is an exciting finding of retrospective analysis of LPP patients which is a common concern among Indian patients. We have seen efficacy of JAK inhibitors in resistant alopecia areata cases in one study. The only limitation factors with respect to JAK inhibitors is the cost as of now.

ARTICLE 60

Randomized Controlled Trial on a PRP-like Cosmetic, Biomimetic Peptides Based, for the Treatment of Alopecia Areata

Rinaldi F, Marzani B, Pinto D, et al. Randomized controlled trial on a PRP-like cosmetic, biomimetic peptides based, for the treatment of Alopecia Areata.
J Dermatolog Treat. 2018;4:1-6.

Abstract

Alopecia areata (AA) is a nonscarring autoimmune hair disorder characterized by loss of hair. In this randomized double-blinded, placebo and active-controlled, parallel group study, the authors have studied the efficacy of a cosmetic product (named TR-M-PRP plus) comprising biomimetic peptides specific for hair growth mimicking platelet-rich plasma (PRP) composition for the treatment of AA. The subjects were treated for 3 months with evaluation done at the end of the study and 1 month after end of study. The evaluation was done for hair growth using Severity of Alopecia Tool (SALT) score. These products showed a statistically significant clinical improvement in SALT score after 3 months of therapy, compared to baseline.

COMMENT

In this study, authors have used biotechnologically designed platelet-rich plasma (PRP)-like cosmetic for treatment of alopecia areata (AA), which was used as an alternative to autologous PRP. The study was a randomized double-blinded, placebo and active-controlled, parallel group study. Sixty subjects with AA of both sexes, aged between 18 and 60 years, were enrolled.

The enrolled subjects were randomly divided into two groups—group I and group II, which included 30 AA patients in each and were treated with TR-M-PRP plus and placebo, respectively. Biomimetic peptides included were—copper tripeptide-1, octapeptide-2, oligopeptide-20 and acetyl decapeptide-3. Lactoferrin, lactoglobulin and melatonin were also included as an anti-inflammatory, adenosine triphosphate (ATP) stimulator and circadian rhythm regulator agents, respectively. Both groups applied the product twice a week (15 mL) for 3 months.

The patients were followed up and digital photos were taken three times at the randomization visit (baseline T0), at the end of treatment period visit at month 3 (T1, 90 days), and at the follow-up visit, one month after treatment end (T2, 120 days).

Alopecia areata grade was assessed according to Severity of Alopecia Tool (SALT) score (S0 = no hair loss; S1 <25% hair loss; S2 = 25–49% hair loss; S3 = 50–74% hair loss;

S4 = 75–99% hair loss; and S5 = 100% hair loss). Percentage of hair regrowth and change in the SALT baseline score were assessed to look for the efficacy of TR-M-PRP plus. Hair regrowth was graded into six grades: A0 = no change or further loss of hair; A1 = 1–24% regrowth; A2 = 25–49% regrowth; A3 = 50–74% regrowth; A4 = 75–99% regrowth; A5 = 100% regrowth.

Of total 60 subjects, 37 were men and 23 were women with mean age 54.32 years and mean of 4.35 symmetrically distributed patchy hair loss and had the last relapse 1–2 years before (mean 1.2). Percentage scalp hair regrowth was assessed based on absolute change in the baseline SALT score for all the patients. Mean value of the absolute change in SALT score was 18.30 and 8.49 for group I and II, respectively. After 3 months of treatment (T1), the mean values were 57.07% for group I and 27.96% for group II. At T2, a significant ($p < 0.0001$) improvement was found for group I (62.01% vs. 28.89% in group II).

In group I, 53.33% cases showed complete regression (A5 grade), 13.33% showed partial regression, but this result was not considered relevant as 33.34% of subjects from group I who showed no response at all. Only 3.33% of population of group II reported a complete regression. No adverse effects were reported in both groups.

The synthesis of biotechnological compound mimicking growth factors opens to novel therapeutic approaches. In this study, all 30 subjects enrolled and treated with TR-M-PRP plus showed significant improvement of SALT score. The results showed the application of biomimetic peptides prolongs the anagen phase (probably acting on Wnt/β-catenin pathways and via exosomes stimulation) and reduces the telogen phase by immunological control, leading to decrease in the hair loss in AA.

Many biomimetic peptides are available but authors have selected mix of peptides which mimic autologous PRP and avoids its limitations like cost, interpersonal variation, invasiveness of the procedure and reported side effects.

Key Messages

- *In treatment of AA, biotechnologically designed PRP-like cosmetic could represent a valid and safer alternative to autologous PRP*
- *Oligopeptide-20 is supposed to increase the synthesis of collagen and glycosaminoglycans by acting as an enzyme inhibitor*
- *Copper tripeptide-1 is a powerful anti-inflammatory agent, stimulates angiogenesis and counteracts hair loss through the stimulation of stem cells increasing hair follicle size*
- *Octapeptide-2 promotes the migration of stem cells and their progeny to the base of the follicle and acts on angiogenesis*
- *Acetyl decapeptide-3 is a basic-fibroblast growth factor (b-FGF) biomimetic which promotes skin regeneration and hair development*
- *Lactoferrin, potent anti-inflammatory agent counteracts inflammation mechanisms of AA*
- *Lactoglobulin is helpful for stimulating ATP production and mitosis*
- *Melatonin regulates hair growth by gene regulation.*

ARTICLE 61

Tofacitinib (Selective Janus Kinase Inhibitor 1 and 3): A Promising Therapy for the Treatment of Alopecia Areata: A Case Report of Six Patients

Shivanna CB, Shenoy C, Priya RA. Tofacitinib (selective Janus kinase inhibitor 1 and 3): a promising therapy for the treatment of alopecia areata: a case report of six patients.
Int J Trichology. 2018;10(3):103-7.

Abstract

Alopecia areata (AA) is a chronic autoimmune disorder characterized by patchy or complete loss of hair from scalp, beard, eyebrows or rarely even body hair. The study was done to show the effectiveness of oral tofacitinib in alopecia univeraslis. Six patients diagnosed with alopecia universalis (AU)/alopecia totalis (AT) duration of disease 6 months to15 years refractory to other treatments were selected and were started on oral tofacitinib 5 mg twice daily up to 10 mg bid and were followed up every 4 weeks and further for 6 months to assess relapse. The efficacy was assessed by hair regrowth using photographic assessment, Severity of Alopecia Tool score, and physical examination. All our six patients showed a dramatic response to oral tofacitinib without significant side effects.

COMMENT

In this study, authors have described the efficacy of tofacitinib in alopecia areata (AA). Six patients diagnosed with alopecia universalis (AU)/alopecia totalis (AT) refractory to immunosuppressants and with rapidly progressing disease were selected. They were evaluated with complete hemogram, liver function test, renal parameters, ultrasound abdomen, chest X-ray, and Mantoux test and also vaccinated for herpes zoster before initiating therapy. All the patients were previously treated with oral corticosteroid or various immunosuppressive like cyclosporine, azathioprine.

The patients were started with oral tofacitinib 5 mg bid for 4 weeks later, and the dose was increased up to 10 mg bid with mean treatment duration of 3–6 months. Therapy was continued till complete regrowth of hairs. Among these patients, initial regrowth was first seen over the eyebrows and beard followed by the scalp. All patients were under remission till 4 months after stoppage of therapy. One patient had relapsed with loss of eyebrows after 2 months of stoppage of drugs. The only side effects observed was acneiform eruptions in two patients.

Tofacitinib is a Janus kinase (JAK) inhibitor (jakinibs) which are a group of drugs that inhibit the JAK family of enzymes interfering with the JAK-STAT signaling pathway. Tofacitinib is a selective targeted kinase inhibitor that it mainly inhibits JAK3, which blocks the upregulation of interferon (IFN)-gamma in CD8+ lymphocytes. Therapeutically, antibody-mediated blockade of IFN-γ, IL-2 or IL-15 receptor have shown to prevent AA disease development, by reducing the accumulation of CD8(+) NKG2D(+) T-cells in the skin and the dermal IFN response in a mouse model. Systemically administered tofacitinib causes pharmacological inhibition of JAK family protein tyrosine kinases, thus reducing downstream effects of the IFN-γ and γc cytokine receptors, and prevents the development of AA. There is an interruption of the feedback loop, and the hair follicles are able to return to anagen. Tofacitinib was initially FDA approved for the treatment of rheumatoid arthritis.

Side effects of jakinibs are anemia, thrombocytopenia and neutropenia due to JAK2 inhibition. There is a report of deranged lipid profile in rheumatoid arthritis patients taking tofacitinib. Other serious adverse effects are bacterial and fungal infections. There are reports of reactivation of TB and herpes zoster in patients during Phase 3 trials. Further studies are required to establish the drug safety profile and long-term side effects.

Key Message
- Tofacitinib a JAK-3 inhibitor is showing promising result in the treatment of severe form of alopecia areata.

ARTICLE 62

Efficacy of Diphenylcyclopropenone in Alopecia Areata: A Comparison of Two Treatment Regimens

Nowicka D, Maj J, Konsur AJ, et al. Efficacy of diphenylcyclopropenone in alopecia areata: a comparison of two treatment regimens.
Postepy Dermatol Alergol. 2018;35(6):577-81.

Abstract
A prospective study comprising 39 patients with alopecia areata (AA) was conducted to assess the efficacy of a topical diphenylcyclopropenone (DPCP) based on the intensity, duration and number of exacerbations of AA and to compare the efficacy of two treatment regimens. Group A was treated at weekly intervals and group B at 3-week intervals. After 6 months' therapy, hair

regrowth greater than 50% was observed in 21 patients, while worsening, no regrowth or regrowth of less than 50% was seen in 18 patients. Regrowth exceeding 50% of initial loss was observed in 12 out of 17 patients with baseline hair loss less than 50%, in nine out of 22 patients with severe alopecia and in four out of nine patients with alopecia totalis. Both groups showed significant improvement with higher efficacy in group B (54%) than group A (46%).

COMMENT

Contact allergens are a well-known treatment option in alopecia areata (AA). Diphenylcyclopropenone (DPCP) is opted when more than 50% of hair loss is present. It acts by antigenic competition causing T-cell response switch from Th1 to Th2 and the reduction of follicular inflammation in AA. The authors have conducted a prospective study comprising 39 patients with AA (23 women and 16 men, aged 14-1 years old (mean age: 39.7 years) to assess the efficacy of a topical DPCP based on the intensity, duration and number of exacerbations of AA; comparing two different application regimens for patients with AA (between a weekly application and an every 21 days application). Severity of AA was assessed based on the Severity of Alopecia Tool (SALT) and a composite scoring done. Accordingly, cases were graded: S0 – no hair loss; S1 – hair loss <25%; S2 – hair loss of 25-49%; S3 – hair loss of 50-74%; S4 – hair loss of 75-99%; and S5 – total scalp hair loss.

A stock solution of 2% DPCP was prepared by dissolving DPCP powder in acetone and diluted on demand to obtain the following concentrations: 0.00001%, 0.0001%, 0.001%, 0.01%, 0.05%, 0.1%, 0.5%, 1% and 1.5% solution. In incrementing doses (starting from 0.00001%) preparation was applied on affected areas until an erythematous reaction lasting for at least 2 days was obtained. Group A had applications on day 1, day 14 and every 7 days thereafter; group B – on day 1 and every 21 days. Treatment efficacy evaluated by two independent dermatologists, photography and dermoscopic documentation was done (3 Gen DERMLITE CAM).

The mean hair loss at baseline was 54.3%. S1 group had eight patients, S2, S3 and S5 had nine patients displaying alopecia totalis and S4 had four patients. After 6 months of treatment, overall 21 patients showed hair regrowth greater than 50% while worsening, lack of regrowth or regrowth of less than 50% was seen in 18 patients. In 17 patients with baseline hair loss <50%, regrowth exceeding 50% of initial loss was observed in 12 patients, while it was below 50% in five of them. In 22 patients with severe alopecia (>50%), regrowth exceeding 50% occurred only in nine cases. In S5 patients, regrowth exceeding 50% was observed in four cases. In 16 patients from group A, mean response was 46%, worsening, lack of regrowth or regrowth of less than 50% was observed in eight patients, and hair regrowth greater than 50% was observed in eight patients. In 23 patients from group B mean response rate was 54%, worsening, lack of regrowth or regrowth of less than 50% was observed in 10 patients, while hair regrowth greater than 50% was observed in 13 patients. Regrowth greater than 50% was observed in three from group A and four from group B in patients with baseline hair loss below 25%; two in patients with total hair loss at baseline. Thus, group B achieved a significantly better outcome. Spearman rank correlation coefficient confirmed that patients with less initial hair loss responded better to treatment (r = 0.6). The efficacy of DPCP was confirmed in patients with different severities of AA. Transient enlargement of neck lymph nodes was observed as prominent side effect in the study.

The authors have proposed a novel regimen of DPCP application which is more effective than the commonly used weekly application. However, results were not correlated with the length of the disease or the number of exacerbations.

Key Messages
- The DPCP is a good therapeutic option, especially in extensive, treatment-resistant AA patients
- The DPCP regimen proposed by authors looks practical and ease. Still, DPCP therapy has potential place in treatment of resistant AA or extensive nature.

ARTICLE 63

Efficacy of Oral Tofacitinib in the Treatment of Lichen Planopilaris

Sallee BN, Bordone LA, Christiano A. Efficacy of oral tofacitinib in the treatment of lichen planopilaris. *J Invest Dermatol. 2018;138(5):S83.*

Abstract
Lichen planopilaris is a chronic inflammatory disorder affecting hair follicles resulting in their destruction and causing cicatricial alopecia. Timely treatment of this condition helps to restore hair growth in affected individuals. The authors have treated eight patients with oral tofacitinib, which resulted in improvement of lichen planopilaris severity score between 30% and 90%.

COMMENT

There is no proven first-line medicine for the management of lichen planopilaris. Various reports are published with many immunomodulatory medicines. Treatment of this disfiguring condition in the early stages is required to prevent extensive permanent hair loss. Use of Janus kinase (JAK) inhibitor tofacitinib in alopecia areata is already established. The same authors here have treated 8 patients of lichen planopilaris with oral tofacitinib successfully. No adverse effects were reported, and flare up was noticed when the drug was withdrawn.

Recent research and developments in regulatory pathogenesis of follicle growth has shed much light on JAK pathway and Wnt signaling pathway. It is also of importance that much light has seen thrown on the JAK pathway in pathogenesis of alopecia areata and cicatricial alopecia. JAK inhibitor molecules were basically used for rheumatoid arthritis and ankylosing-spondylitis also showed improvement in hair disorders. At this point of time drugs are too expensive for routine prescription and require a well-controlled study.

Key Message

- The JAK inhibitor tofacitinib has emerged as another treatment option for lichen planopilaris, for early control of the disease thus preventing permanent hair follicle loss.

ARTICLE 64

Isotretinoin Treatment for Folliculitis Decalvans: A Retrospective Case-series Study

Aksoy B, Hapa A, Mutlu E. Isotretinoin treatment for folliculitis decalvans: a retrospective case-series study. *Int J Dermatol. 2018;57(2):250-3.*

Abstract

This retrospective record-based study aims at determining the most effective dose and duration of oral isotretinoin monotherapy for achieving remission in folliculitis decalvans (FD) patients. As per the medical records based information, authors suggest that isotretinoin at a dose of ≥0.4 mg/kg/day should be given for ≥3 months to minimize the likelihood of relapse.

COMMENT

Folliculitis decalvans (FD) is one of the primary cicatrising alopecia involving vertex and occipital area causing a lot of distress in patients. Though antibiotics are being used as first line of treatment the drawback is quick relapse following discontinuation of treatment. Thus requiring long-term antibiotics.

In this study, 39 male patients clinically diagnosed as FD and treated with oral isotretinoin monotherapy were retrospectively analyzed. The analysis showed that oral isotretinoin monotherapy is an effective treatment with long-lasting result. The results are seen after 3 months of treatment with less relapse chances. The recommended dosage is ≥0.4 mg/kg/day for a minimum period of ≥3 months to achieve long-term remission. Hyperlipidemia and dryness were the common side effects observed.

> **Key Messages**
> - *Isotretinoin can be an effective therapeutic option in the management of FD*
> - *Given at a dose of ≥0.4 mg/kg/day for a minimum of 3 months reduces the chance of relapse*
> - *The isotretinoin dose in cases of resistant cases of FD should be above the dose used for acne. Generally recommended dose of isotretinoin for FD should be 40 mg/day low doses leads to early relapse.*

ARTICLE 65

Clinical Studies Evaluating Abametapir Lotion, 0.74%, for the Treatment of Head Louse Infestation

Bowles VM, VanLuvanee LJ, Alsop H, et al. Clinical studies evaluating abametapir lotion, 0.74%, for the treatment of head louse infestation.
Pediatr Dermatol. 2018;35(5):616-21.

Abstract

Background: There is a need for better control of head louse infestations. Abametapir is an inhibitor of metalloproteinases critical for louse survival and egg development. The efficacy of abametapir lotion, 0.74%, was assessed for its ability to clear head louse infestations after a single application.

Methods: Two randomized, double-blind, multicenter and vehicle-controlled studies were conducted in subjects aged 6 months and older to compare the effectiveness of abametapir lotion versus vehicle control for eliminating head louse infestations without nit combing. Abametapir lotion was applied to dry hair for 10 minutes on day 0 and then rinsed with water. The primary endpoint was the proportion of index subjects (youngest household member with ≥3 live lice at screening) in the intent-to-treat population who were louse free at all follow-up visits through day 14. Older household members with one or more live lice at screening were designated as nonindex subjects and treated as per the index subject within their household.

Results: In the intent-to-treat population (index subjects, n = 216), 81.5% of subjects treated with abametapir lotion were louse free through day 14 after a single treatment, versus 49.1% with vehicle (p <0.001). For the combined index and nonindex population (n = 704), 85.9% were louse free through day 14 in the abametapir group, versus 61.3% in the vehicle group (p <0.001). The most frequently reported adverse events were erythema (4%), rash (3.2%) and skin burning sensation (2.6%).

Conclusion: Abametapir lotion, 0.74%, was effective at clearing active head louse infestations through day 14 in subjects aged 6 months and older. All adverse events (including one serious but unrelated to study drug) resolved uneventfully.

COMMENT

Head louse infestation is one of the common infestations in school going children. Most of the times these head louse infestations are treated with over-the-counter (OTC) products containing synergized pyrethrin or synthetic pyrethroid (permethrin). Rampant and irregular use of these agents has led to the emergence of resistance to these agents. At the same time, all these agents having nervous system of the louse as the target site contribute to the resistance. So the search for new target is the need of the hour.

Evidence from many studies have shown that proteases, including metalloproteinases, are involved in the process of louse egg hatching and metal-chelating agents are shown to inhibit this protease activity in vitro studies. Abametapir is a one such metalloproteinase inhibitor targeting metalloproteinases critical to the development of adult lice. Abametapir 0.74% was applied over dry scalp and massaged into the scalp and hair, working from the hairline at the back of the neck to the end of the hair. It was left for 10 minutes and then rinsed off. During follow-up at day 1, 7 and 14, therapeutic end point was absence of live lice and safety end point included adverse events and evaluations for skin, scalp and ocular irritation.

Abametapir demonstrated statistically significant cure rate as compared to vehicle with greater percentage of index subjects achieving treatment success. These studies hypothesized that abametapir can provide effective and safe therapy in the management of head louse. The studies also hypothesized that a single application is sufficient. Patient compliance is also better thus avoiding irregular treatment which in turn prevents emergence of resistance.

Safety analysis showed minimal erythema, rash, burning sensation and discoloration which subsided within 7 days. No other serious adverse effects were reported.

Key Messages

- Abametapir 0.74% lotion is safe and effective therapeutic modality in the treatment of head louse
- As metalloproteinases required for egg hatching are the new targets, single application is sufficient and chances of resistance are remote
- There are several treatment options available for louse infestation. The resistance developed and need for frequent application limits their usage. The new drug abametapir with different mechanism of action promises to be unique, still needs second application once eggs hatch out nymphs. The drug acting on all stages of development especially on egg stage is still elusive.

ARTICLE 66

Apremilast for Moderate Hidradenitis Suppurativa: Results of a Randomized Controlled Trial

Vossen ARJV, van Doorn MBA, van der Zee HH, et al. Apremilast for moderate hidradenitis suppurativa: results of a randomized controlled trial.
J Am Acad Dermatol. 2019;80(1):80-8.

Abstract

This study was conducted to evaluate the short-term efficacy of apremilast in hidradenitis suppurativa (HS). Twenty patients with moderate HS were prescribed apremilast and placebo in the ratio of 3:1 for a duration of 16 weeks. Fifty-three percent of patients on apremilast showed clinical response as opposed to none in the placebo group at the end of 16 weeks. Apremilast treated group had a lower abscess and nodule count. Most common side effects noted were headache and gastrointestinal symptoms.

COMMENT

Hidradenitis suppurativa (HS) is a chronic inflammatory disease presenting with painful, itchy, deep-seated inflamed nodules, abscess and sinus tracts predominantly over the axilla, groin and perianal area. The incidence is slightly more common in females and causes a lot of morbidity and social handicap in the affected patients.

Currently, the therapies include antibiotics, especially the tetracycline group, rifampicin and clarithromycin. The only approved biologic is adalimumab. Apremilast is a phosphodiesterase 4 inhibitor which modulates a variety of inflammatory mediators. It has been used extensively in psoriasis and psoriatic arthritis.

The authors have included moderate cases of HS, as apremilast is proven to be less efficacious than biologic agents used for psoriasis. Patients were treated with oral apremilast 30 mg twice a day after randomization. Patients were screened at 2, 4, 8, 12 and 16 weeks after starting therapy. At the end of 6 weeks 53.3% of patients achieved significant improvement in lesions, improvement was seen as early as 2 weeks. The results were comparable to those achieved with adalimumab in moderate hidradenitis. The onset of clinical response was much faster in the HS group as compared to the studies with psoriasis which may be explained by the differences in pharmacodynamic patterns. About 30 mg twice daily of apremilast was well tolerated by most of them and side effects were rated as mild-to-moderate. The short-term safety profile of apremilast has been established by various studies. Most common side effects noted were headache, diarrhea, nausea and common cold. No serious adverse reports were reported. All the side effects had resolved within 8 weeks of completing the treatment. Only one patient discontinued the study due to severe muscle and joint pain.

Hidradenitis suppurativa is a chronic disease, and there are no treatments which offer permanent cure. Apremilast has the advantage over antibiotics and biologics. Continuous use of antibiotics can induce bacterial resistance. With biologics, continuous lab monitoring and subcutaneous administration are required. Apremilast is the drug under evaluation for various inflammatory disorders which has prostaglandin E as a component. PDE is one of the enzyme in the inhibitory cascade, HS being a chronic inflammatory disorder is one more indication for the usage of this drug.

Key Message

- Apremilast is a PDE4 inhibitor which has multiple roles in the inflammatory cascade. A dose of 30 mg twice daily has been used extensively in psoriasis. This study has shown significant clinical improvement in patients with moderate HS. Apremilast appears to be a promising new molecule in the treatment armamentarium of HS.

ARTICLE 67

Apremilast for Moderate Hidradenitis Suppurativa: No Significant Change in Lesional Skin Inflammatory Biomarkers

Vossen ARJV, van der Zee HH, Davelaar N, et al. Apremilast for moderate hidradenitis suppurativa: no significant change in lesional skin inflammatory biomarkers.
J Eur Acad Dermatol Venereol. 2019;33(4):761-5.

Abstract

The authors in the previous article have shown clinical improvement in moderate hidradenitis suppurativa (HS) with apremilast. This study also included the change of inflammatory markers in lesional skin after treatment. At baseline two punch biopsies were taken, one from erythematous indurated lesional skin and the other from nonaffected skin from the same anatomic location. Biopsies were repeated at 4 and 16 weeks from the neighboring sites of previous biopsies. Statistically significant changes in inflammatory markers were not noted after treatment, though there was significant clinical improvement. However, S100A12 and IL-17A levels showed significant decrease in response to treatment.

COMMENT

Hidradenitis suppurativa (HS) is a chronic skin condition with limited treatment options. The previous article has shown significant improvement clinically in patients receiving apremilast 30 mg twice a day for 16 weeks. The authors in the same study have evaluated the inflammatory biomarkers before and after treatment. After sampling, biopsies were split whereby one half was processed for mRNA analysis of the biopsy, representing the in vivo gene expression, and the other half was cultured for ex vivo protein analysis. Though 17 proteins showed a baseline increase, there was no significant difference in levels in marker expression after treatment. Out of the 17 genes analyzed, there was no significant downregulation of mRNA also. S100A12 (calgranulin C, ENRAGE) is a proinflammatory, calcium-binding antimicrobial protein that is overexpressed in various inflammatory skin diseases and stimulates the cells to produce IL-17A. Though there was a decrease in S100A12 and IL-17A levels, it was not significant. Due to the fluctuating nature of the disease, the spontaneous improvement of few lesions in the placebo group could explain the reduction in inflammatory markers in the placebo group.

Key Messages

- *This translational study investigating apremilast in moderate HS did not detect statistically significant changes in important inflammatory markers in lesional skin compared with placebo over 16 weeks of treatment, despite positive clinical findings*
- *By analysis these two studies, where clinical improvement is not substanderdized by the change in inflammatory biomarkers. These appear to be some other mechanism of action of apremilast to be explored which brings improvement in HS.*

ARTICLE 68

A Case of Isotretinoin Therapy-refractory Folliculitis Decalvans Treated Successfully with Biosimilar Adalimumab (Exemptia)

Shireen F, Sudhakar A. A case of isotretinoin therapy-refractory folliculitis decalvans treated successfully with biosimilar adalimumab (Exemptia).
Int J Trichology. 2018;10(5):240-1.

Abstract

Folliculitis decalvans is a chronic disorder of the scalp characterized by recurrent episodes of pus discharge and scarring. The various treatment options are isotretinoin, antibiotics like doxycycline or minocycline. Inspite of the various available therapies there is no permanent cure for it. It causes severe disability due to the recurrences. Here, the authors report a case of folliculitis decalvans treated successfully with adalimumab biosimilar.

COMMENT

The authors have treated a chronic case of recurrent folliculitis with adalimumab biosimilar. The patient had been suffering from 5 years and had been treated in the past with multiple cycles of isotretinoin. The lesions would resolve during therapy and recur immediately within one week of stopping the medications. The authors initiated a course of doxycycline and terbinafine for 2 weeks with topical clindamycin and fluocinolone. Post this the patient was treated with isotretinoin again for another 6 weeks. As there was no improvement with any of these, the patient was prescribed adalimumab biosimilar 80 mg on week 0 and week 2 and then 40 mg on weeks 3, 4, 6, 8, 10, 12, 14 and 16. The patient was weaned off from isotretinoin 2 weeks after initiation of biosimilar. No recurrences have been noted since then, however, the patient is still on a monthly dose of biosimilar. No adverse events were noted.

Key Message

- Adalimumab or its biosimilar can be considered for management and to maintain patient of folliculitis decalvans in remission.

ARTICLE 69

Turmeric Tonic as a Treatment in Scalp Psoriasis: A Randomized Placebo-control Clinical Trial

Bahraini P, Rajabi M, Mansouri P, et al. Turmeric tonic as a treatment in scalp psoriasis: a randomized placebo-control clinical trial.
J Cosmet Dermatol. 2018;17(3):461-6.

Abstract

The present article is a prospective trial to explore the potential therapeutic effects of turmeric in scalp psoriasis. In comparison to the placebo group, turmeric tonic markedly decreased the erythema, scaling and induration of lesions [Psoriasis Area and Severity Index (PASI) score] in the treated group and improved the patients' quality of life (p-value <0.05).

COMMENT

Turmeric (*Curcuma longa* L.), is a well-acclaimed spice worldwide, known to have anti-inflammatory, antimicrobial, antifibrotic, antioxidant, hypocholesterolemic and antineoplastic properties due to its active component *curcumin (diferuloylmethane)*. Its inhibitory activity on potassium channels in T cells is reported to play a key role in psoriasis. Topical vitamin D analogs and corticosteroids are well-established first-line treatments for scalp psoriasis along with tar-based preparations, tacrolimus, dithranol and salicylic acid. However, curcumin is found to bind to 5-LOX, xanthine oxidase, thioredoxin reductase, COX-2, p-glycoprotein, GST, PKA, PKC, cPK, PK, Ca^{2+}-dependent protein kinase (CDPK), and glutathione and suppress phosphorylase kinase (PhK) activity thereby brings about resolution of psoriatic lesions. Elevated PhK activity is associated with depletion of glycogen granules in active psoriasis. It also correlates with the presence of the specific markers during proliferation, including expression of PCNA/Ki-67 antigen, presence of parakeratosis, thin elongated rete pegs, and suprapapillary thinning and vice versa during resolution. Curcumin being a potent PhK inhibitor induces clinical remission of psoriatic lesions.

The present study is a placebo-controlled, double-blind, randomized study done to evaluate the usefulness of turmeric tonic in mild-to-moderate scalp psoriasis. Forty patients aged 18-75 years, with 2-week washout of topical treatment, and/or 1-month washout with systemic treatment were recruited, allocated by block random allocation (with a 1:1 allocation) into two parallel groups. The case group received turmeric tonic twice a day and the control group applied placebo in the same manner; followed up every 3 weeks for the test period of 9 weeks and 4 weeks post-trial. The clinical efficacy of the treatment was evaluated by

Psoriasis Area and Severity Index (PASI) scores and Dermatology Life Quality Index (DLQI) questionnaire, during and after treatment. Generalized irritation, stinging or allergic reaction to formulation at the treatment sites were prompt indicators of treatment stoppage.

Thirty patients completed the study (about 50 participants in each group; 40 patients of scalp psoriasis randomly allocated in these groups). A uniformity in demographic factors and disease intensity between the intervention and control group has been maintained. Mean age in the interventional group was 29 years (M:F = 9:6), in the control group it was 44 years (M:F = 12:3). The diagnosis duration of >1 year was predominantly seen in both groups, also positive family history (73.3% in the interventional group; 46.7% in control group), and body involvement in 66.7% of the interventional group and 46.7% of control group has been observed. Turmeric tonic was found to be more effective than the placebo in decreasing the PASI score from the beginning to the end of the study, (p <0.05) and also the patient's quality of life (p <0.05). Mean erythema, scaling and thickness scores before, during, and after treatment were important parameters that showed response with no adverse effects. Observations of PASI at 3, 6 and 9 weeks in both groups have shown a steady decline in PASI; at week 9 PASI median was 0.3 in the interventional group; 0.4 in the placebo group. Similarly, DQLI improved much better in the interventional group compared to placebo.

The study appears to be reasonably well conducted. The benefits of curcumin are known since ages but by the observation made, different concentration and formulation curcumin should be given emphasis in future evaluation.

However, the study also showed that the emollient effect of placebo decreased the PASI scores in the control group.

Limited sample size and short post-trial follow-up warrants more clinical trials to confirm the efficacy of turmeric. Standardized topical formulation and vehicle also need to be established, as topical microemulgel preparation by Sarafian G et al. and 1% curcumin gel formulation by Thomas AE et al. have been tried with satisfactory results.

Key Messages

- Curcumin is a potent, selective and noncompetitive phosphorylase kinase inhibitor; reduce PhK levels and decreases the expression of proinflammatory cytokines and growth factors IL-6 and IL-8 in psoriatic lesions
- It can be used alone or in combination with other treatments as an effective and safe therapeutic option.

ARTICLE 70

An Open-label, Observational Study Evaluating Desoximetasone Topical Spray 0.25% in Patients with Scalp Psoriasis

Bagel J, Nelson E. An open-label, observational study evaluating desoximetasone topical spray 0.25% in patients with scalp psoriasis.
J Clin Aesthet Dermatol. 2018;11(5):27-9.

Abstract
This is an open-label, observational study evaluating the efficacy, tolerability and patient satisfaction of desoximetasone 0.25% spray in patients with scalp psoriasis.

COMMENT

Twenty patients with plaque psoriasis of the scalp were enrolled in this 16-week study. They used desoximetasone spray 0.25% twice daily for 4 weeks, followed by twice-daily application on two consecutive days per week for an additional 12 weeks. Subjects also applied the study material to other areas affected by plaque psoriasis, excluding the face, groin and axillae.

The Investigator's Global Assessment (IGA) scale score of scalp involvement, using a 5-point (0-4) scale that recorded overall disease severity based on average scores for erythema, induration and scaling of affected areas made at each visit. The IGA scale used was 0 = clear, 1 = almost clear, 2 = mild, 3 = moderate and 4 = severe. Psoriasis Scalp Severity Index (PSSI) and scalp surface area (SSA) were also calculated. Rapid onset of action across all efficacy parameters, with significant improvements seen as early as week 4 after initiation of treatment, thus optimizing initial control. The physician global assessment (PGA), body surface area (BSA), BSA × PGA, scalp IGA and PSSI were reduced from baseline by 55%, 51%, 63%, 65% and 82.4%, respectively. After 4 weeks, desoximetasone 0.25% spray was decreased from twice-daily application to twice-daily application on two consecutive days per week from week 4 through week 16. Improvements from baseline were maintained at week 16. At week 16, PGA and scalp IGA were reduced from baseline by approximately 50%. Additionally, PSSI was reduced by 63.4% at week 16.

The level of efficacy combined with the convenience and the use of a patient-preferred spray vehicle suggest that this is an effective therapy for scalp psoriasis. A larger, randomized, controlled trial is necessary to corroborate and extend these results.

Key Messages

- Due to better efficacy and convenient use, spray is the preferred vehicle for the scalp, male chest and other hair-bearing locations, as well as when there is extensive skin involvement
- Foam-based steroids preparation are the first choice for scalp psoriasis but stability of foams in a country like India is a big challenge. Till the ideal foam is brought clinicians have to depend on sprays and lotion.

ARTICLE 71

Prolonged Skin Retention of Clobetasol Propionate by Bio-based Microemulsions: A Potential Tool for Scalp Psoriasis Treatment

Langasco R, Tanrıverdi ST, Özer Ö, et al. Prolonged skin retention of clobetasol propionate by bio-based microemulsions: a potential tool for scalp psoriasis treatment.
Drug Dev Ind Pharm. 2018;44(3):398-406.

Abstract

Novel effective and cosmetically acceptable formulations are needed for the treatment of scalp psoriasis, due to the poor efficacy of the current products. The challenge in developing safe, efficient and convenient delivery systems for this drug was addressed in the present work by formulating clobetasol propionate loaded W/O microemulsions (MEs). Pseudoternary phase diagrams were constructed by using a combination of biocompatible and biodegradable excipients. Characterization studies demonstrated that selected MEs had suitable technological features such as being Newtonian fluids, possessing low viscosity and high thermodynamic stability. Photomicrographs showed a significant alteration of the skin structure after treatment with MEs, and a preferential concentration of these in the stratum corneum and epidermis. These data, together with ex vivo permeation results, suggested an enhanced topical targeted effect due to an increased drug retention efficacy in the upper skin layers, as desired. Moreover, the bio-based excipients selected could contribute to the healing of the psoriatic scalp. In this way, the improvement of clobetasol efficacy is combined with the useful properties of the ME components and with environmental safety.

COMMENT

Psoriasis is a common papulosquamous disorder affecting entire body, scalp and extremities. Scalp psoriasis can have highly variable presentation. Treatment included topical corticosteroid, vitamin D analog and phototherapy. Among topical steroid clobetasol-17-propionate (CP) has been proven to be the most potent steroid. It is available as solutions, shampoos and foams. These formulations are safe for short term (up to 4 weeks) due to its topical side effects (skin atrophy and telangiectasia). This article reviews new topical vehicles for CP delivery to overcome the side effects of the drug.

Microemulsions (MEs) are formed instantaneously when interfacial tension between oil and water is reduced close to zero. In this study, various MEs ingredients (ME1 and ME2) were chosen and tested for safety and acceptability of the formulation. Olive oil and 2-propanol were chosen as for ME1 and IPM and ethanol were selected for ME2 as oil phase and cosurfactant, respectively. ME2 had higher water content and low shear stress, and viscosity compared to ME1 leading to better penetration compared to ME1.

Stratum corneum, lipid bilayer prevents penetration of drugs. Many studies with different formulation tried to disrupt or weaken the stratum corneum to improve skin delivery. Nanocarriers and lipid-based delivery systems have been used to increase skin transportation by improving drug solubilization in the formulation, drug partitioning into the skin and by fluidizing the skin lipid.

Key Message

- W/O microemulsion appeared to deeply alter scalp psoriasis with higher drug concentration enhancement in the various upper skin strata. These MEs are bio-based formulations with promising controlled CP delivery system for the treatment of scalp psoriasis. This formulation is noninvasive, can be applied easily with enhance patient compliance. These MEs improves topical delivery and skin retention efficacy of CP with prolong drug release and simultaneously reduce the corticosteroid side effects.

ARTICLE 72

Scalp Psoriasis: Report of Efficient Treatment with Secukinumab

Pistone G, Tilotta G, Gurreri R, Curiale S, Bongiorno MR. Scalp psoriasis: report of efficient treatment with secukinumab. *J Dermatolog Treat. 2018:1-10.*

Abstract

Psoriasis is a chronic inflammatory skin disease affecting 2–3% of the population in the world. The scalp is the most common, and frequently the first site of disease involvement. Occasionally it may be the only localization of psoriasis. Treatment of scalp psoriasis is often unsatisfactory, due to limited available topical therapy and reduced efficacy of some systemic drugs. Biologic therapies are recommended for severe psoriasis, resistant to topical treatment, but evidence from randomized controlled studies is lacking regarding effectiveness on scalp-localized lesions. Several clinical studies have shown the efficacy of secukinumab on plaque psoriasis, and some encouraging experience suggest the use in difficult sites such as the scalp; this article reports effective treatment, with secukinumab, of a series of patients with plaque and scalp psoriasis.

COMMENT

Ten adult patients (six males and four females) with moderate-to-severe plaque psoriasis located in the scalp were recruited for treatment with secukinumab. Skin and scalp psoriasis localization were assessed at baseline, at week 6 and at week 12. Scalp involvement was evaluated using the Psoriasis Scalp Severity Index (PSSI) [(score range: 0-72)]. The extent and severity of skin involvement was done by Psoriasis Area Severity Index (PASI) and the body surface area (BSA). Secukinumab was administered subcutaneously with the dosage of 300 mg once weekly at weeks 0, 1, 2, 3 and 4 for induction, and then every 4 weeks for maintenance therapy, up to week 12.

The average age was 44.6 years; 35% of patients were overweight (average body mass index of 28.7). PSSI mean score was 48.8 (range 16-72) at baseline. About 50% of patients exhibited plaque psoriasis with severe involvement of more than 50% of the skin surface, with an overall average PASI of 38.6 and an average BSA of 47%.

Improvement of scalp psoriasis was seen as early as week 4 and PSSI mean score was reduced to 32.3 (range 8-52) at week 6. 60% of patients had achieved at least 70% improvement in the PSSI score and 30% showed at least a 75% improvement. Similar improvement was observed for skin psoriasis, at week 6, the PASI mean score was reduced to 11.4 and the BSA at 9.5%. Patients achieved complete remission at week 12 and 6; the remaining four patients achieved an improvement of PSSI and PASI score of 90%. Mean PSSI was 1.2 (range 2-4). Reduction in the PSSI was comparable to the response obtained on the skin.

In the study, rapid improvement of scalp psoriasis was appreciated by the authors proposing secukinumab in chronic and recurrent cases especially multiple site psoriasis and of unresponsive localizations like scalp. However, efficacy and safety profile of secukinumab in scalp psoriasis need more controlled trials.

Key Messages

- Secukinumab is a human monoclonal IgG1 antibody, selectively binds and neutralizes IL-17; key player in the pathogenesis of plaque psoriasis
- We have treated more than 100 cases of chronic plaque psoriasis with secukinumab using standard dosage and protocol. We found extremely good response in almost all patients response sets in as early as second dosage of secukinumab with complete clearance in most of our patients by 5th dose. Recurrence does occur after stopping but only in few cases. Long-term remission of scalp psoriasis is an added benefit in majority of patients
- Secukinumab is one of the choices in extensive and treatment resistant cases of scalp psoriasis.

ARTICLE 73

Efficacy and Safety of 308 nm Excimer Lamp in the Treatment of Scalp Psoriasis: A Retrospective Study

Rattanakaemakorn P, Phusuphitchayanan P, Pakornphadungsit K, et al. Efficacy and safety of 308-nm excimer lamp in the treatment of scalp psoriasis: a retrospective study.
Photodermatol Photoimmunol Photomed. 2019;35(3):172-7.

Abstract

Scalp psoriasis poses a therapeutic challenge due to the hindrance caused by hair. This retrospective study was done to evaluate the efficacy, safety, and effective dosage of 308 nm excimer light in the treatment of scalp psoriasis. This study included 20 patients with scalp psoriasis who received 308 nm excimer light. Patients were evaluated with Psoriatic Scalp Severity Index (PSSI) before and after treatment. Around 11 patients responded to treatment at the end of 10 sessions. This modality could be considered as an alternative or adjuvant treatment for scalp psoriasis.

COMMENT

Up to 80% of patients with psoriasis report scalp lesions. Psoriasis of the scalp has been considered to cause a significant impact on patients' quality of life (QOL). Scalp psoriasis is considered as easy to recognize and relatively easy to treat in its normal presentation but at times becomes difficult when does not respond to regular treatment or there is contraindication to systemic treatment.

This study demonstrates the successful use of the 308 nm monochromatic excimer light (MEL) device in the treatment of scalp psoriasis. The treatment achieved a statistically significant reduction of Psoriatic Scalp Severity Index (PSSI) (12 to 4.5) and at the end of treatment period the itch score (median itch score 3.5 to 0.5). There was rapid clearing of the psoriatic lesions with a starting dose of 500 mJ/cm^2. With no serious side effects, most patients well tolerated dose increment of 20% at each visit.

The increase in intensity of monochromatic 308 nm light causes T-cell apoptosis due to attack of the target lesional T-cells, this has been proposed as the mechanism of action proposed for MEL.

Monochromatic excimer light provides greater fluency with deeper skin penetration, attributed to increased irradiance in comparison to conventional phototherapy. The modality requires fewer treatment sessions and lower cumulative dose to obtain the same effect. On comparison with conventional phototherapy, remission duration of MEL-treated lesions was greater.

This study reports the efficiency of MEL therapy in decreasing itching in scalp psoriasis patients. MEL may reduce lesional T-cells that release certain cytokines and decrease the psoriatic lesions IL-31 levels, associated with pruritus.

The various study limitations are that it has relatively small number of patients and it is a retrospective study. Further, to overcome these limitations, prospective randomized controlled trials (RCTs) in greater number of patients can be conducted.

Key Messages

- *This study successfully demonstrates the use of excimer 308 nm lamp as adjuvant treatment in psoriasis of the scalp*
- *In comparison to conventional phototherapy and excimer laser, the advantages of excimer light are it being specific on target, wider irradiation field, greater ability to penetrate skin, shorter therapeutic time, lower power density and accumulative dose requirement and fewer treatment sessions.*

ARTICLE 74

Trichotillomania Treated with N-acetylcysteine

Kılıç F, Keleş S. Trichotillomania treated with N-acetylcysteine.
Psychiat Clin Psych. 2018.

Abstract

Trichotillomania (TTM) is a disorder characterized by repetitive hair pulling resulting in hair loss and it is usually difficult to treat with a chronic course of illness. Currently, the selective serotonin reuptake inhibitors (SSRIs) are the most frequently prescribed drugs for adults with

TTM. Various studies and case reports give mixed results. Therefore, the treatment effectiveness of SSRIs remains uncertain. There is a growing interest regarding the use of glutamatergic agents in obsessive compulsive disorder (OCD) and obsessive compulsive spectrum disorder. Here, we report an 18-year-old female patient with TTM, who was successfully treated with glutamate modulator N-acetylcysteine.

COMMENT

An 18-year-old high school student experienced recurrent, irresistible urges to pull out hair from her scalp every day and spent almost an hour on hair pulling, more during stressful times, while watching television or studying, nearly for a year. She had developed visible hair loss at temporal areas, and used a bandanna during the day. Her behavior had affected her quality of life. She felt sad, pessimistic, anxious, especially after a hair pulling act. Her symptom severity was assessed with beck anxiety inventory (BAI) and beck depression inventory (BDI), and scores were 17 and 20, respectively. A final diagnosis of Trichotillomania (TTM) was confirmed.

After initial treatment with escalated dose of fluoxetine 40 mg/day, hair pulling decreased, but the time spent, hair loss and accompanying thoughts were not affected noticeably. Later risperidone was started 0.5 mg/day and was unsuccessful. With a daily dose of 1,200 mg, water-soluble form N-acetyl cysteine (NAC) therapy was initiated. After 3 weeks, all the urges and behaviors related to hair pulling had stopped dramatically. There were no symptoms of anxiety and depression or any side effects. At 2 months after initiating treatment, her hair loss in the temple region of her scalp improved markedly as well and NAC was discontinued. During 6-month follow-up, no further symptoms related to hair pulling were observed and she has been able to continue her daily activities.

Selective serotonin reuptake inhibitors are usually considered first-line treatment option for obsessive compulsive disorder (OCD). NAC, a mucolytic, functions as a glutamate modulator. In Trichotillomania (TTM), increase in glutamate levels results in exacerbated oxidative stress and more severe OCD symptoms. However, NAC decreases extracellular glutamate concentrations in nucleus accumbens and reduces compulsive behaviors in TTM. Drug is also found to be well tolerated at dose range of 1,200–2,400 mg/day. However, further studies are needed to establish a treatment regimen and evaluate its long-term effectiveness.

Key Messages

- The NAC modulates the glutamatergic system and improves TTM symptoms. It alleviates TTM symptoms by achieving lower brain glutamate levels
- A lot of reports are available regarding usage of NAC in TTM. Most of them are case reports that outline benefits of NAC. It is worthwhile considering this option in treating TTM.

ARTICLE 75

Treatment of Seborrheic Dermatitis: A Comprehensive Review

Borda LJ, Perper M, Keri JE. Treatment of seborrheic dermatitis: A comprehensive review.
J Dermatolog Treat. 2019;30(2):158-69.

Abstract

Seborrheic dermatitis (SD) is a chronic, recurring inflammatory skin disorder that manifests as erythematous macules or plaques with varying levels of scaling associated with pruritus. The condition typically occurs as an inflammatory response to *Malassezia* species and tends to occur on seborrheic areas, such as the scalp, face, chest, back, axilla and groin areas. SD treatment focuses on clearing signs of the disease; ameliorating associated symptoms, such as pruritus and maintaining remission with long-term therapy. Since the primary underlying pathogenic mechanisms comprise *Malassezia* proliferation and inflammation, the most commonly used treatment is topical antifungal and anti-inflammatory agents. Other broadly used therapies include lithium gluconate/succinate, coal tar, salicylic acid, selenium sulfide, sodium sulfacetamide, glycerin, benzoyl peroxide, aloe vera, mud treatment, phototherapy, among others. Alternative therapies have also been reported, such as tea tree oil, *Quassia amara* and *Solanum chrysotrichum*. Systemic therapy is reserved only for widespread lesions or in cases that are refractory to topical treatment. Thus, in this comprehensive review, we summarize the current knowledge on SD treatment and attempt to provide appropriate directions for future cases that dermatologists may face.

COMMENT

Management of Seborrheic dermatitis (SD) should focus not only on clearing signs and symptoms, but also to maintain long-term remission. Topical therapy is commonly used, but systemic therapy may be needed in case of widespread lesions or when refractory to topical therapy.

Topical antifungals are usually the first-line of therapy as they reduce the *Malassezia* burden and subsequently the inflammation. Topical ketoconazole 2% shampoo and cream has been shown to be more effective than steroids with much lesser adverse effects. 2% miconazole, 1% clotrimazole and 1% terbinafine are as effective as ketoconazole. Sertaconazole cream is effective in facial SD. 1% ciclopirox olamine has shown more than 75% improvement during 3rd to 4th week.

Though mild to mid potent steroids are effective in clearing the signs and symptoms of SD, their prolonged use results in side effects. Steroids clear symptoms faster than pimecrolimus, but relapses are also faster than pimecrolimus. Nonsteroidal anti-inflammatory agents are efficacious and well tolerated. Piroctone olamine and climbazole are effective with little or no side effects. Topical bisabolol cream when applied twice daily for 30 days has shown significant improvement in erythema, desquamation, and pruritus compared to baseline. Glycyrrhetinic acid and lactoferrin have also be shown to be effective nonsteroidal anti-inflammatory agents.

Tacrolimus ointment has the advantage of no side effects like skin atrophy and telangiectasia as compared to steroids. It is as effective as steroids and sertaconazole. It does cause burning, itching and irritation during the initial days of application. It is better to be used for long-term maintenance once the initial erythema and scaling is controlled. Pimecrolimus, being a cream preparation, produces better cosmetic acceptability, generally well tolerated than tacrolimus. It has shown to be as effective as hydrocortisone and ketoconazole. In addition, tacrolimus is in ointment base and can cause occlusion leading to exacerbation of disease initially; a lotion-based preparation is better and well tolerated.

Shampoos containing coal tar and salicylic acid induce exfoliation, stimulation of epidermal renewal, and antimicrobial activities against *Malassezia ovalis*. Selenium sulfide shampoo has the same effectiveness as ketoconazole shampoo; however, ketoconazole appears to be better tolerated. Narrow-band ultraviolet B (NBUVB) therapy has been shown to be very effective for severe SD with occasional moderate erythema postexposure.

Systemic therapy is reserved for very severe SD. Oral itraconazole, terbinafine and oral fluconazole are the main systemic therapies used for treating SD, although prednisone (0.5 mg/kg/day) taken over the course of 15 days and low-dose oral isotretinoin (0.1 mg/kg/day every other day) over the course of 6 months have proven effective in treating moderate-to-severe SD.

Studies involving the use of oral biotin for treating SD have had conflicting results. Topical 4% nicotinamide gel has been shown to have 75% efficacy in treating the symptoms.

Key Message

- Topical therapeutic modalities include antifungal and anti-inflammatory agents, selenium sulfide, metronidazole, lithium gluconate/succinate, and phototherapy. Systemic therapy is indicated in severe refractory cases. The treatment should be individualized according to each patient's profile
- The therapeutic choice in SD should be toward nonsteroidal anti-inflammatory and antifungal agents as possible to avoid dependency on steroids, which in long-term are detrimental to skin health.

Section 4: Therapeutic Trichology (Procedural Intervention)

ARTICLE 76

The Effectiveness of Adding Low-level Light Therapy to Minoxidil 5% Solution in the Treatment of Patients with Androgenetic Alopecia

Faghihi G, Mozafarpoor S, Asilian A, et al. The effectiveness of adding low-level light therapy to minoxidil 5% solution in the treatment of patients with androgenetic alopecia.
Indian J Dermatol Venereol Leprol. 2018;84(5):547-53.

Abstract

Low-level light therapy (LLLT) stimulates hair growth in both men and women but lacks controlled clinical trials. This study compares the effectiveness of adding LLLT to topical minoxidil in the treatment of androgenetic alopecia (AGA) in 50 patients of 17–45 years age group for one year. The case group received topical minoxidil 5% + LLLT twice per day. The control group received only topical minoxidil 5% and placebo laser comb. The mean hair density and diameter were higher in the case group than the control group. LLLT can be definitely be an add-on therapy.

COMMENT

Androgenetic alopecia (AGA) is the most common type of alopecia, in genetically-predisposed individuals, often caused by androgens such as testosterone and its derivatives. Treatment of AGA includes the use of topical minoxidil, the administration of Finasteride tablets and hair transplantation. LLLT is a new technique for stimulating hair growth in men and women. It stimulates anagen phase re-entry in telogen hair follicles, prolong the duration of anagen phase, increase rates of proliferation in active anagen hair follicles and prevent premature catagen development. This was a randomized, double-blind, controlled study which was conducted to carry out a comparative assessment of the effectiveness of adding LLLT to minoxidil topical solution for the treatment of alopecia in patients presenting to skin clinics in Isfahan, Iran. The case group received topical minoxidil 5% solution twice per day plus 2-3 20-minute sessions of LLLT (10–50 mW power and a 785-nm wavelength) per week for 24 weeks. The controls received only topical minoxidil 5% and were given a laser comb system that was switched off to act as a placebo. Hair analysis was done using trichogram. The percentage of recovery from AGA was similar in both groups 3 months after the intervention; however, compared to the controls, the case group revealed a significant increase in this percentage at 6, 9 and 12 months after the intervention. The mean hair diameter was significantly higher in the cases compared to the controls only 12 months after the intervention and not before. The stimulating effect of low-level light on hair growth can be achieved through a direct or indirect increase in the proliferative intra matrix activity of the epithelial hair follicles. This study overcame the weaknesses of previous studies on the subject and is considered a scientific clinical trial of the effectiveness of LLLT in the treatment of AGA.

> **Key Messages**
> - Low-level light therapy is a new technique for stimulating hair growth through a direct or indirect increase in the proliferative intra matrix activity of the epithelial hair follicles
> - It improves the percentage of recovery in AGA cases and provides patient satisfaction.

ARTICLE 77

Effectiveness of Low-level Laser Therapy in Lichen Planopilaris

Fonda-Pascual P, Moreno-Arrones OM, Saceda-Corralo D, et al. Effectiveness of low-level laser therapy in lichen planopilaris.
J Am Acad Dermatol. 2018;78(5):1020-3.

Abstract
This study analyzes the effectiveness of low-level laser therapy (LLLT) in lichen planopilaris (LPP). The article showed that the LLLT can be a newer therapeutic modality in the management of LPP. However, because of its small sample size and lack of histopathology data author recommends further study in large scale.

COMMENT

Lichen planopilaris (LPP) is a chronic lymphocytic mediated inflammatory condition resulting in permanent destruction of hair follicles. The condition being progressive requires long-term treatment. Low-level laser therapy (LLLT) is emerging as a treatment modality in many inflammatory conditions. This study evaluates the potential usefulness of LLLT in patients with lichen planopilaris. LLLT has demonstrated to increase peroxisome proliferator-activator receptor gamma (PPAR-γ) expression in murine models of inflammation.

The study involved clinically and histologically confirmed cases of LPP. Lichen Planopilaris Activity Index (LPPAI), with a final score from 1-10 was used as a clinical variable before and after treatment. Specific areas were marked and videodermatoscopic analysis of scalp was done to evaluate trichoscopic images and to assess inflammation (perifollicular erythema and hyperkeratosis), terminal and global hair follicle thickness.

Patients were started on LLLT with devices with high-powered unfocused 246 red LED, at a wavelength of 630 nm and a fluence of 4 J/cm^2 were used 15 minutes daily for 6 months.

At the end of 6 months, there was global reduction of symptoms, erythema and perifollicular hyperkeratosis in all patients. It also showed a mean decrease of 0.87 in LPPAI-score after 6 months of therapy (p = 0.012). There was an increase in terminal hair thickness after 3 months (p = 0.018) as well as after 6 months (p = 0.035).

To conclude LLLT is an emerging treatment for LPP requiring large scale studies.

Key Messages

- Low-level laser therapy is an emerging alternative therapy in the management of LPP
- LLLT devices are available in different variants, some also combine multiple wavelengths. Before putting patients on LLLT physician should be aware of power and wavelengths. Number of sessions and frequency of LLLT depends on the device used but practical experience with regard to above parameters is the key to success
- It reduces follicular inflammation by increasing peroxisome proliferator-activator receptor gamma (PPAR-γ) expression.

ARTICLE 78

Low-level Light-minoxidil 5% Combination versus Either Therapeutic Modality Alone in Management of Female Patterned Hair Loss: A Randomized Controlled Study

Esmat SM, Hegazy RA, Gawdat HI, et al. Low-level light-minoxidil 5% combination versus either therapeutic modality alone in management of female patterned hair loss: a randomized controlled study.
Lasers Surg Med. 2017;49(9):835-43.

Abstract

This article analyzes the efficacy of low-level light therapy (LLLT) in the management of female pattern hair loss (FPHL) as a monotherapy and in combination with minoxidil also in comparison with topical minoxidil 5% alone. It showed that combination of LLLT with minoxidil works better than monotherapy alone.

COMMENT

Female pattern hair loss (FPHL) is the most common form of hair loss in women. The FDA approved therapeutic modalities for FPHL are topical minoxidil and more recently low-level light therapy (LLLT). Low-level laser therapy is postulated to have efficacy in promoting hair growth in both men and women with androgenetic alopecia (AGA) and FPHL, respectively. The probable mode of action of LLLT could be due to its ability to stimulate epidermal stem cells in the hair follicle bulge, induce the follicles into anagen phase, initiate protein synthesis that triggers cell proliferation and migration, and tissue oxygenation. It also induces vasodilation thus increasing blood flow to the scalp, thus improving patients with FPHL.

In the current study, subjects were randomly allocated into three groups with one group receiving topical minoxidil 5% lotion, second group receiving LLLT with laser diodes and 30 LEDs, 655 nm red laser with output <5 mW, CW and LED wavelength ranging from 650 nm to 670 nm for 25 minutes on alternate day and third group receiving combination of above two for 4 months duration.

Clinical assessment of each group separately at the end of 4 months showed significantly better results in third group receiving combination therapy ($p < 0.001$).

Ultrasound biomicroscopy (UBM) at the end of 4 months showed significant increase in the number of hair follicles in both second and third groups and also the hair follicles induced by the combined therapy were observed at a deeper dermal level when compared to other modalities. Regarding folliscope finding among the different groups, a significant increase in the mean hair density was detected in all groups. Dermoscopy showed marked reduction in the diversity of hair diameter in the three groups with no significant difference noted between the three groups.

To conclude low-level laser is an effective and safe tool for the treatment of FPHL. It is comparable with a slight upper hand over minoxidil 5%. The combination of both techniques seems to be preferable over monotherapy.

Key Messages

- *Low-level laser is an effective and safe tool for the treatment of FPHL*
- *It can be combined with topical minoxidil for optimum results*
- *Several studies have proved the efficacy of LLLT in FPHL as well as AGA. The key to success lies in choosing optimal wavelength diode preferably between 600 nm and 800 nm, frequency of treatment and duration of each LLLT exposure.*

ARTICLE 79

Platelet-rich Plasma for the Treatment of Female Pattern Hair Loss: A Patient Survey

Laird ME, Lo Sicco KI, Reed ML, et al. Platelet-rich plasma for the treatment of female pattern hair loss: A patient survey. Dermatol Surg. 2018;44(1):130-2.

Abstract

Androgenetic alopecia (AGA) in women, also known as female pattern hair loss (FPHL), is the most common cause of hair loss, affecting up to 50% of women over the course of their lifetime, and is known to progress with age and menopause. Although topical minoxidil and oral finasteride are being used but they have their own drawbacks. Platelet-rich plasma (PRP) is a novel method for treating various types of alopecia. Clinical studies in animal models have demonstrated PRP's efficacy as there is significant improvement in hair density and stimulation of hair growth.

COMMENT

Platelet-rich plasma (PRP) therapy is a new modality of treatment bridging the gap of medical and surgical mode of treatment for hair loss. This anonymous voluntary survey was sent through email, to assess the patient satisfaction. Females between 18 years and 90 years of age, who had undergone one or more PRP therapy prior to 6 months, were included in the study. About 76% of them completed the survey. All patients had tried other therapies like minoxidil, finasteride etc. A majority of patients were satisfied (58%), with 65% of satisfied patients reporting either "marked" or "exceptional" improvement. Most common subjective manifestations of improvement were hair feeling/looking fuller or thicker to the patient or others (94%) and less shedding (61%). Frequently reported side effects were swollen face/forehead and painful scalp lasting for 3 days. Patients were more satisfied if they reported new hair growth as a manifestation of improvement, did not report any adverse reactions, or required two or fewer treatments to see improvement. This study supports a growing body of literature that PRP is a promising new therapy in the treatment of FPHL.

Key Messages

- Platelet-rich plasma is a new modality of treatment for FPHL
- There are very few adverse effects like forehead swelling and painful scalp, that are transient
- Somehow the data available so far regarding PRP therapy is not conclusive with respect to efficacy. However patient's satisfaction rate appears to be high in all studies.

ARTICLE 80

The Effect of Autologous Activated Platelet-rich Plasma Injection on Female Pattern Hair Loss: A Randomized Placebo-controlled Study

Tawfik AA, Osman MAR. The effect of autologous activated platelet-rich plasma injection on female pattern hair loss: A randomized placebo-controlled study.
J Cosmet Dermatol. 2018;17(1):47-53.

Abstract

This study evaluates the efficacy and safety of autologous platelet-rich plasma (PRP) in the treatment of female pattern hair loss (FPHL) in 30 patients who were randomly assigned to receive autologous PRP injection in a selected area, and other area was injected with placebo. They were assessed both subjectively and objectively at the end of 6 months. There was not only significant improvement in hair density and hair thickness but also the hair pull test became negative in PRP-injected areas in 25 patients with photographic improvement in hair volume and quality with high patient satisfaction. Hence PRP can be an alternative cost-effective treatment with minimal morbidity in FPHL.

COMMENT

Female pattern hair loss (FPHL), or androgenetic alopecia (AGA) in females, is the most common type of hair loss affecting women characterized by shortening of the anagen phase and miniaturization. Thinning and widening of the area of hair loss occur on the central part of the scalp. The treatment modalities vary from medical treatment such as minoxidil, 5α-reductase inhibitors, to surgical modality as hair transplantation. Platelet-rich plasma (PRP) is a new promising modality of treatment with no adverse effects. The basic idea behind PRP injection is to deliver high concentrations of growth factors to the scalp, with the hope of stimulating hair regrowth.

This prospective randomized placebo-controlled study was conducted on 30 patients to evaluate the efficacy and safety of autologous PRP in the treatment of FPHL. Patients, who had received topical or systemic treatments for hair loss in the previous 3 months, were excluded. Patients who were pregnant or those with a history of keloids, malignancies, bleeding disorders, and thyroid dysfunction were also excluded. Laboratory tests were done to rule out other causes of hair loss. This was a split half study with one area randomly receiving PRP and the other area placebo. Four treatments were given for each patient, with an interval of 1 week between the sessions. Patients were followed up at 6 months after the last session. For PRP separation, 10 mL of blood was collected which was subjected to double centrifugation, after which PRP was mixed with calcium gluconate 1:9 ratio before injecting, using an insulin syringe.

Global photography, hair pull test, patient's satisfaction scale, and standardized phototrichograms were used to evaluate the results. PRP-injected sites showed an overall improvement in hair density and thickness, as lanugo-like hair became thicker, normal hair. Moreover, a significant reduction in hair loss was noticed by patients. Additionally, there was a statistical significant difference between PRP and placebo areas ($p < 0.005$) regarding both hair density and hair thickness at 6-month follow-up. Patients were satisfied with a mean result rating of 7.1 on a scale of 1–10 without noting any remarkable adverse effects.

The growth factors contained in platelets of blood plasma include platelet-derived growth factor (PDGF), transforming growth factor-b, vascular endothelial growth factor (VEGF), epidermal growth factor, and connective tissue growth factor (FGF). When platelets become activated, these growth factors are released and promote differentiation of stem cells into hair follicle cells through the upregulation of transcriptional activity of beta-catenin. PRP injection for FPHL is a simple, cost-effective and feasible treatment option with an excellent safety profile.

Key Messages

- PRP contains platelet-derived growth factor (PDGF), transforming growth factor-beta, vascular endothelial growth factor (VEGF), epidermal growth factor, and connective tissue growth factor (FGF) which promote differentiation of stem cells into hair follicle cells through the upregulation of transcriptional activity of beta-catenin
- PRP is prepared by double centrifugation followed by activation with calcium gluconate
- PRP improves hair density and thickness and reduces hair loss.

ARTICLE 81

A Comparative Study of Microneedling with Platelet-rich Plasma Plus Topical Minoxidil (5%) and Topical Minoxidil (5%) Alone in Androgenetic Alopecia

Shah KB, Shah AN, Solanki RB, et al. A comparative study of microneedling with platelet-rich plasma plus topical minoxidil (5%) and topical minoxidil (5%) alone in androgenetic alopecia.
Int J Trichology. 2017;9(1):14-8.

Abstract

This study evaluates the efficacy of microneedling with platelet-rich plasma (PRP) plus topical minoxidil (5%) versus topical minoxidil (5%) alone in androgenetic alopecia (AGA), III to V vertex

(Norwood–Hamilton scale), in 50 men between 18 years and 50 years. These patients were randomly divided into group A – 25 patients: topical minoxidil (5%) alone and group B – 25 patients: topical minoxidil (5%) + microneedling with PRP. All patients were assessed at baseline and end of 6 months by both patient and physician based on standardized seven-point scale. There was a significant improvement ($p < 0.05$) in both patients' assessment and investigator's assessment in topical minoxidil, microneedling and PRP group, and hence this combination can be safe, effective and a promising for managing AGA.

COMMENT

Yet another study rolling out the benefit of PRP. The concept of wounding and resultant release of growth factors to promote healing is a well-established fact. The authors on these principles have conducted this study combining microneedling with PRP. The comparative results between groups satisfactorily prove the benefit of combining PRP with microneedling and topical minoxidil. If one more group consisting of only microneedling with minoxidilwould have given even more comparative analysis whether improvement is because of PRP or microneedling. Our understanding at this point of time for all these kind of treatments are in nascent stage and probably we are on the way of developing some evidence which ultimately may lead to standardization of protocols of PRP treatment.

Key Message

- *Microneedling with platelet-rich plasma is a safe adjuvant option for AGA. It would have added more light if another group consisting of only microneedling with minoxidil was evaluated to prove the efficacy of microneedling or PRP over both.*

ARTICLE 82

Comparison of the Efficacy of Homologous and Autologous Platelet-rich Plasma for Treating Androgenic Alopecia

Ince B, Yildirim MEC, Dadaci M, et al. Comparison of the efficacy of homologous and autologous platelet-rich plasma (PRP) for treating androgenic alopecia.
Aesthetic Plast Surg. 2018;42(1):297-303.

Abstract

The aim of this study was to compare increase in hair density, average number of platelets, complications, preparation and duration of application in the treatment of androgenetic alopecia (AGA) using a-PRP (activated autologous platelet-rich plasma), n-PRP (nonactivated autologous PRP), and h-PRP (homologous PRP). There were three groups who received n-PRP a-PRP, and h-PRP, respectively at 1, 2 and 6 months. The hair density was counted before and after each session. The conclusion was an increase in density of hair was more with h-PRP group than autologous PRP group.

COMMENT

This study was done to see the effectiveness of h-PRP (homologous platelet-rich plasma) for androgenetic alopecia (AGA) compared with autologous PRP. The study had three groups with 20 male patients each in the age group of 25–35 years with Norwood type 2–4 baldness grade. Patients with anemia, any thyroid hormone, iron or vitamin B12 deficiency were excluded.

The n-PRP (nonactivated autologous PRP) for group 1 was prepared with Young Cell 10 mL PRP kit. A 40 mL blood was subjected to a single spin at 3,000 rpm for 15 minutes. At the end, 4–5 mL of PRP was obtained for each patient. The a-PRP for group 2 was prepared with Truecell 10 mL PRP kit. After the first centrifugation, the plasma and buffy coat portions of the centrifuged blood were transferred to the kit with calcium chloride and centrifuged at 2,000 rpm for 5 minutes. At the end, 4–5 mL of PRP was obtained for each patient. The h-PRP for group 3 was obtained from pooled platelets prepared at the blood center.

The PRP injections were performed at a 1.5–2.5 mm deep intradermal area with 0.05–0.1 mL/cm^2 using an insulin injector. The digital photographs were taken before and after each injection and were evaluated using NEO Image Analysis Software.

The mean platelet counts from the complete blood count were 281,000, 264,000 and 232,000 µ/L, respectively in 3 groups. At 2, 6 and 12 months after the first treatment, the increase in hair density was calculated as 11.2%, 26.1% and 32.4%, respectively, in group 1; 8.1%, 12.5% and 20.8%, respectively, in group 2; and 16.09%, 36.41% and 41.76%, respectively, in group 3. The study showed an increase in hair density in all groups by second month. An increase in hair density was significantly greater in group 1 than in group 2 and more so in group 3 than in both groups among all controls ($p < 0.05$).

The authors feel that an increase in hair density count is more with h-PRP groups compared to autologous PRP group may be due to an increasing platelet counts as well as more growth factors in h-PRP. The h-PRP has 4–5 donor growth factors which act synergistically to give more hair density counts.

The authors also found out that results with n-PRP were better than a-PRP because of lower levels of insulin-like growth factor 1 (IGF-1) and vascular endothelial growth factor (VEGF) after activation in the kit.

The advantages of h-PRP are its easy preparation, availability of high platelet counts in microliters and more PRP obtained.

The h-PRP is prepared from blood centers, so there is no additional time for preparation. It only needs to be injected which takes approximately 10 minutes on average. Thus there is significant time saving as compared to autologous PRP.

Key Message

- Authors propose that the homologous PRP is as and more effective than autologous PRP in treatment of androgenetic alopecia with the advantage of time saving and free from hassles of autologous PRP preparation.

ARTICLE 83

A Meta-analysis on Evidence of Platelet-rich Plasma for Androgenetic Alopecia

Giordano S, Romeo M, di Summa P, et al. A Meta-analysis on evidence of platelet-rich plasma for androgenetic alopecia. *Int J Trichology. 2018;10:1-10.*

Abstract

Platelet-rich plasma (PRP) has been used increasingly in the treatment of androgenetic alopecia (AGA). This study was a systematic literature search to identify the effects of PRP in terms of increase in the number of hair as well as thickness of the hair. Seven studies which were done with PRP on one side versus control on the other side were included. There was significant increase in the hair density per cm² in the PRP injected area with a significant increase in hair thickness.

COMMENT

Platelet-rich plasma (PRP) is an autologous product obtained by centrifugation of patients own venous blood. PRP contains 3–8 times the platelet concentration as compared to normal peripheral blood. On activation, the platelets are degranulated releasing a variety of growth factors. The complex interaction of growth factors and tissue proteins is believed to stimulate angiogenesis and hair growth. PRP has been used for management of androgenetic alopecia (AGA) extensively.

In this study, the authors have reviewed seven studies involving 194 patients to observe the effects of PRP injections on the scalp for the treatment of AGA. Studies which used quantitative methods to check the outcomes compared with a control were included in the study. The primary outcome used to assess the effect of PRP was the change in the number of hair per cm². Changes in hair cross-section and thickness percentage were used as secondary outcomes. Few studies have used the contralateral side as control, and others have used patient groups.

Among the cases reviewed significant increase in the number of hair per cm² was observed in the PRP groups. Also, significant difference in the hair thickness diameter was noted. There is no standardized method of preparation of PRP. This might explain the differences in the outcomes and product composition. There is no standardization yet regarding the amount of PRP to be injected, the frequency of injections and the number of injections. PRP has also shown promising results in post-transplant cases.

Key Message
- As PRP is an autologous product, the risk of transmission of infections is minimal. It has emerged as a safe, effective, can be administered in outpatient and affordable treatment for androgenetic alopecia. It is used mainly along with topical minoxidil and as adjuvant post hair transplantation.

ARTICLE 84

Platelet-rich Plasma on Female Androgenetic Alopecia: Tested on 10 Patients

Starace M, Alessandrini A, D'Acunto C, et al. Platelet-rich plasma on female androgenetic alopecia: tested on 10 patients. *J Cosmet Dermatol.* 2019;18:59-64.

Abstract
This article analyzes the efficacy and safety of platelet-rich plasma (PRP) injections in female androgenetic alopecia (AGA). PRP has therapeutic effect on hair density and hair diameter improvement in those refractory to medical line of management.

COMMENT

Androgenetic alopecia (AGA) is the most common genetically determined progressive noncicatricial alopecia affecting up to 80% of men and 50% of women. Under the influence of dihydrotestosterone, hair follicles undergo miniaturization with short anagen phase. In female pattern hair loss (FPHL), there will be diffuse thinning of crown with intact frontal hair line (Ludwig pattern). In FPHL only FDA approved treatment is 2% minoxidil twice a daily or 5% foam once daily and oral anti-androgen, which can be used either alone or with combination. Medications need to be continued for longer time for good results. There is a need for adjuvant therapy. Recently, platelet-rich plasma (PRP) injection has been advocated as a potential adjuvant therapeutic technique for AGA.

This study was done to evaluate the safety and the efficacy of injection PRP those who were not responding to topical and oral medications for FPHL. Total of five injection sites were chosen using a standardized scalp grid (vertex, parietal, central and frontal area). At each point, 1 cc was injected every 2 weeks for four sessions under topical anesthesia. "V" point is calculated by the intersection of the mid-sagittal line and the coronal line connecting both tips of the tragus of the patient. Other point is taken 6 cm toward the frontal line and 6 cm toward the vertex. The parietal injections were performed at 4 cm from the "V" point toward the tip of the tragus. Results were evaluated as clinical improvement by pull test, global photographs, and TrichoScan at weeks 9, 12 and 24. At follow-up vellus hair showed significant reduction and increase in the hair diameter which was evident in the front and the central area.

Platelet-rich plasma is an autologous plasma containing 2-3 times increased concentration of platelets from its baseline value. The actual mechanisms of action is still under debate and standardization PRP with respect to optimal concentration, methods of preparation, frequency of treatment and long-term sustainability is yet to be validated. It induces the proliferation of dermal papilla cells and prevents the apoptosis by inducing the increase in Akt and Bcl-2 expression. Furthermore, anagen phase is prolonged by increased expression of FGF-7 (fibroblast growth factor-7) and it suppresses inflammatory cytokines.

Key Message

- Though injection PRP is an adjuvant treatment in female androgenetic alopecia, especially in patients refractory to standard approved therapies such as minoxidil and antiandrogens, studies are still required to standardize the technique, frequency of treatments for effective results and optimal duration of the therapy to maintain the results.

ARTICLE 85

A Randomized Controlled Study of the Effect of Intralesional Injection of Autologous Platelet-rich Plasma Compared with Topical Application of 10% Minoxidil in Male Pattern Baldness

Goyal V, Mathur D, Nijhawan M. A randomized controlled study of the effect of intralesional injection of autologous platelet rich plasma (PRP) compared with topical application of 10% minoxidil in male pattern baldness. *JDA Indian Journal of Clinical Dermatology.* 2018;1:26-7.

Abstract

A randomized double blinded control trial of 105 cases. The cases were divided randomly into three groups; group A [injected with platelet-rich plasma (PRP)], group B (applied 10% minoxidil), and group C was the control group. Patients of group A showed statistically significant increase in their mean hair density showing that PRP has a role in male pattern hair loss.

COMMENT

Androgenetic alopecia (AGA) (male pattern hair loss) is the most common cause of diffuse hair loss characterized by miniaturization of hair follicles. Nonsurgical treatment options are always preferred as first-line of therapy with topical minoxidil being FDA approved while PRP is also showing promising results. PRP essentially contains growth factors which promote tissue repair, angiogenesis (capillary formation), collagen production, and normalization of the follicular unit. PRP contains increased concentration of platelets about 10,00,000 platelets/μL in comparison with normal blood.

The article aims to compare the effect of intralesional autologous PRP and topical 10% minoxidil in the patients of male pattern baldness. A randomized double blinded control trial in 105 cases was done. Three groups—group A (injected with PRP), group B (applied 1 mL of 10% minoxidil twice daily), and group C control group (applied rose water) with 35 patients in each group with similar age and sex profile were considered. Six injections of PRP (0.1 mL/cm^2) were given at an interval of 21 days in all patients. TrichoScan analysis for hair thickness and density was performed at baseline and then performed monthly for 6 months.

In group A, the mean hair thickness increased by 2.9 μm, while in group B and group C it was found to be 2.6 μm and 0.3 μm, respectively. This was not statistically significant. On the contrary, the mean hair density in group A, at baseline and at the end of 6 months, was 100.9 and 121.8 follicular units per cm^2, respectively. In group B, the mean hair density was 98.4 and 106.4 follicular units per cm^2 and group C was 104.2 and 104.9 follicular units per cm^2, respectively. This improvement in patients of group A was statistically significant with respect to increase in their mean hair density. Thus, PRP showed better results in the study in comparison to minoxidil and author's propose it as an important adjunct in treatment options of AGA.

However, in this study, the method of PRP preparation was a single spin technique, 20 mL whole blood sample drawn was centrifuged at the rate of 1,000 rpm for 10 minutes activated with 10% calcium chloride to avoid crystallization of solution and then injected intradermally. Validation of PRP technique needs to be substantiated with further studies to gain more evidence before it is widely advocated.

Contrary to that, this study has used 10% minoxidil which has no evidence and lacks case-control studies. Indications for using 10% minoxidil are not elaborated. One has to have clear cut guidelines to use higher concentration of minoxidil although individual observation from clinicians proposes use of 10% minoxidil for AGA.

Key Message
⊙ Platelet-rich plasma is useful adjunct modality in male pattern hair loss.

ARTICLE 86

Fractional Non-ablative Laser-assisted Drug Delivery Leads to Improvement in Male and Female Pattern Hair Loss

Bertin ACJ, Vilarinho A, Junqueira ALA. Fractional non-ablative laser-assisted drug delivery leads to improvement in male and female pattern hair loss.
J Cosmet Laser Ther. 2018;20(7-8):391-4.

Abstract

Androgenetic alopecia (AGA), also known as male and female pattern hair loss, is a very prevalent condition; however, approved therapeutic options are limited. Fractionated laser has been proposed to assist in penetration of topical medications to the cutaneous tissue. We present four cases of AGA that underwent treatment with a non-ablative erbium glass fractional laser (NAFL) followed by the application of topical finasteride 0.05% and growth factors including basic fibroblast growth factor, insulin-like growth factor (IGF), vascular endothelial growth factor (VEGF), and copper peptide 1%. During all laser treatment sessions, eight passes were performed, at 7 mJ, 3–9% of coverage, and density of 120 mzt/cm^2. A positive response was observed in all of the four patients. Photographs taken 2 weeks after the last session showed improvement in hair regrowth and density. No significant side effects were observed.

COMMENT

Fractionated laser has been proposed to assist in penetration of topical medications to the cutaneous tissue. In this case report, four cases were applied with topical finasteride 0.05% and growth factors including basic fibroblast growth factor, vascular endothelial growth factor (VEGF), insulin-like growth factor (IGF), and copper peptide 1% after NAFL. Improvement in hair regrowth and density was documented by photographs taken 2 weeks after the last session.

Non-ablative fractional lasers applied alone have been shown to be effective in the treatment of hair diseases such as alopecia areata, female and male pattern hair loss as it causes wounding source, increasing blood flow, cytokines and growth factors expression, as well as on stem cell and/or dermal papilla cell stimulation.

In this study, nonablative 1,550 nm fractional erbium glass laser (Fraxel, Solta Medical, Hayward, CA) was used. During all laser treatment sessions, eight passes were performed, at 7 mJ, 3-9% of coverage, and density of 120 mzt/cm^2. No anesthesia was administered and an epidermal cooling device was used during the procedure to reduce the pain. Immediately after laser treatment, all patients received 2 mL of topical finasteride solution 0.05% compounded with distilled water as the vehicle. A 2 mL compounded solution of growth factors, including basic fibroblast growth factor, VEGF, IGF, and copper peptide 1.2%, was also applied topically.

Four cases of patterned alopecia were treated, three were male and one was female patient. After each treatment, all the patients were advised not to apply any other topical medication to their scalp, neither to start any new systemic drug.

A positive response was observed in all of the four patients. Improvement in hair regrowth and density was observed on global photographs taken 2 weeks after the last session when compared to baseline photos. No significant side effects were observed. Large studies are required to further elucidate the mechanism of this improvement.

Key Messages

- *Fractional technique creates an array of microscopic wounds across the surface of the skin as "channels" which enhance penetration of topical agents, such as finasteride and growth factors compound solutions*
- *However, topical finasteride penetration is questionable as transcutaneous absorption is hindered by its molecular weight and size but this study used ablative fractional laser to enhance penetration. Molecular tagging and biopsy for tissue concentration are more authenticated and become evidence-based if done.*

ARTICLE 87

Microneedling for the Treatment of Hair Loss?

Fertig RM, Gamret AC, Cervantes J, et al. Microneedling for the treatment of hair loss?
J Eur Acad Dermatol Venereol. 2018;32:564-9.

Abstract

Microneedling is minimally invasive dermatological procedure which utilizes multiple fine needles to create multiple micropunctures in the skin. It promotes neovascularization, the release of growth factors, and stimulates collagen production. It has been used in a variety of dermatologic diseases, including androgenetic alopecia (AGA) and alopecia areata, among others. This review article summarizes the gist of articles published on microneedling as a treatment option in cases of AGA and alopecia areata.

COMMENT

This article is a review which defines the current literature stand regarding microneedling in the treatment of alopecia. Microneedling has specifically been demonstrated to increase hair regrowth in alopecia due to the release of various growth factors like vascular endothelial growth factor (VEGF), insulin-like growth factor (IGF), basic-fibroblast growth factor (b-FGF), platelet-derived growth factor, epidermal growth factors and activation of the hair bulge with increased expression of Wnt proteins, namely Wnt3a and Wnt10b, all of which are triggered by the wound healing response.

Currently, five prototype roller instruments registered with the FDA. Few of them are for home use and others are for office use. The length of needles varies from 0.13 mm to 1.5 mm. In addition to rollers, there are smaller microneedling devices such as the stamp and pen which are useful for treating small, localized areas of skin and hair.

Dhurat et al. conducted a 12-week, randomized, evaluator-blinded controlled study comparing the results of weekly microneedling sessions used in combination with 5% minoxidil solution applied twice a day for 12 weeks to the twice-daily application of 5% minoxidil alone. Fifty patients were randomly recruited in each group. All subjects had their heads shaved prior to treatment to ensure the same length of hair at baseline. The microneedling group had received weekly sessions for 12 weeks. The outcome of treatment was assessed with hair count after 12 weeks in a predefined area with 1 cm diameter. Patients with microneedling sessions with minoxidil therapy had hair count 91.4 versus control hair count 22.2 ($p = 0.039$).

Another study by Dhurat et al., 6-month, case series of 4 subjects who were resistant to finasteride and minoxidil therapy were treated with 15 microneedling sessions over 6 months, initial weekly 4 sessions, followed by 11 sessions 2 weeks apart in addition to their existing finasteride and minoxidil therapy for AGA. It improved new hair growth by more the 75% in three of four patients and by more than 50% in one of four patients.

Farid et al. conducted a 28-week, randomized, evaluator-blinded, controlled study with 40 patients to the efficacy of PRP was applied in conjunction with microneedling once monthly for 6 months with twice daily 1 mL 5% minoxidil cream for AGA. The outcome was both treatments worked equally by improving hair growth, and patients were equally satisfied but minoxidil worked significantly quicker.

Sasaki presented a case series with 10 patients for the effect of treatment with microneedling combined with PRP for AGA. The outcome was average hair count was 88.3 ± 22.5 prior to treatment, and after PRP microneedling, it was 133.6 ± 13.8 in a 10-mm spot.

Lee et al. published a 5-week, scalp-split, single-blinded, placebo-controlled study where one half of the scalp of each subject was treated with growth factors followed by microneedling and other half was treated with saline and followed by microneedling for AGA. The result showed average hair count was 52.91 ± 10.85 on the treated side of the scalp compared to 45.91 ± 9.98 on the control side of the scalp.

Thus, all studies showed that the use of microneedling in AGA has been found to have positive therapeutic results, particularly when combined with topical minoxidil.

Microneedling and alopecia areata has also been studied by Lee et al. in a 2-week, scalp-split, single-blinded, placebo-controlled study on 6 patients in which microneedling was performed on one half the scalp prior to application of a photosensitizer used in photodynamic therapy and on other half photosensitizer was applied without prior microneedling before photodynamic therapy. There was no hair regrowth in treatment or control group.

Chandrashekhar et al. published a case series of two patients in which topical triamcinolone was applied before and after microneedling for three sessions each 3 weeks apart in alopecia areata. The outcome was excellent restoration of hair growth.

Microneedling in alopecia areata has not shown much efficacy but can be used to augment the delivery of topical steroids for good therapeutic response.

Key Messages

- *There are many publications, case reports, and personal views on microneedling in treatment of alopecia none of the cases series are large enough to prove or disprove the concept. Therapeutic wounding definitely modifies the proliferative aspects of tissue regrowth but to extrapolate it to hair regrowth requires large case series with proper methodology*
- *Microneedling in AGA in various studies have shown a positive response by improving hair regrowth in conjunction with other FDA approved treatment like minoxidil and finasteride*
- *Microneedling in alopecia areata has not shown much encouraging response, but can be used to augment delivery of topical steroid for faster regrowth.*

ARTICLE 88

Intradermal Injections of a Hair Growth Factor Formulation for Enhancement of Human Hair Regrowth – Safety and Efficacy Evaluation in a First-in-Man Pilot Clinical Study

Kapoor R, Shome D. Intradermal injections of a hair growth factor formulation for enhancement of human hair regrowth – safety and efficacy evaluation in a first-in-man pilot clinical study.
J Cosmet Laser Ther. 2018;20(6):369-79.

Abstract

Background: Research has shown the efficacy of hair growth factors in hair regrowth. We describe the intradermal injections of a recombinant, bioengineered hair formulation, containing growth factors, into the scalp skin, for enhancement of hair regrowth and evaluate its efficacy.

Objectives: The objective of this study was to assess the efficacy and safety of the hair growth factor formulation in reducing hair loss and enhancing hair growth.

Materials and Methods: This was an open-label, prospective, single-arm interventional pilot study in which 1,000 patients were given intradermal injections of a hair formulation into the scalp skin. The formulation contains vascular endothelial growth factor, basic fibroblast growth factor, insulin-like growth factor, keratinocyte growth factor, thymosin β4 and copper tripeptide-1 suspended in a sterile injectable vehicle. Intradermal injections of this hair formulation were injected into the scalp once every 3 weeks for a total of eight such sessions. Hair pull test was performed before every session. Videomicroscopic and global images were taken at baseline, fourth session, eighth session, and 2 months after the completion of the eight sessions. Relevant safety assessments through physical examination, questionnaires and appropriate laboratory examination were conducted throughout the study.

Results: Significant reduction in hair fall was seen in 83% of the patients on the hair pull test. Videomicroscopic image evaluation showed that most patients had a decrease in the number of vellus hair, increase in number of terminal hair and increase in shaft diameter. Seventy-five percent of the patients believed that the hair injections were aiding the treatment of their hair loss, and it was also beneficial in posthair transplant patients. At 1 year, a statistically significant increase in total hair count ($p = 0.002$) continued to be seen. Treatment was well tolerated.

Conclusion: Intradermal injections of this hair formulation may be a promising option for treating male as well as female patterns of hair loss.

COMMENT

The most common cause of baldness or hair loss is androgenetic alopecia in which the current surgical, medical and cosmetic interventions are limited in approach and success. There are many growth factors which have been found to stimulate the hair growth cycle. The authors have prepared a bioengineered, recombinant formulation, consisting of a combination of growth factors, administered intradermally, capable of preventing hair loss and stimulating hair growth which consists of vascular endothelial growth factor (VEGF) (human oligopeptide-11), basic fibroblast growth factor (FGF) (human oligopeptide-3), insulin-like growth factor (human oligopeptide-2), copper tripeptide-1, keratinocyte growth factor and thymosin β4. This solution was first tried on mice for safety and efficacy studies.

This is an open-label, prospective, single-arm interventional pilot study, in which 1,000 patients were treated for hair loss. The Indian males and females of age group 20–60 years were included. All patients were having male pattern/female pattern hair loss which did not respond inspite of 1 year or more of treatment with topical minoxidil (2% alone for women) and (5% in men) along with oral 1 mg finasteride. Patients were excluded if they have recent history of starting the treatment or who had recent post-hair transplant hair loss.

The present formulation utilizes an intradermal pharmaceutical formulation which includes the growth factors along with vitamins, minerals, nucleic acids, and amino acids, and diluents. This solution was administered with nappage technique at the intradermal level for 8 sessions, 3 weeks apart in the total volume of 1.5 mL in the affected areas.

Scalp assessment and evaluation was done with hair pull test at each visit with global photographic assessment and videomicroscopic assessment to know the condition of hair growth. There was a significant reduction in hair fall in 83% of the patients when assessed with hair pull test. There was an increase in number of terminal hair as well as an increase in hair shaft diameter and decrease in vellus hair number on videomicroscopic image evaluation. Seventy-five percent of the patients told and believed that hair injections were helping the treatment of their hair loss, and also beneficial in post-hair transplant surgery patients. There was statistically significant increase in total hair count ($p = 0.002$) at the end of 1 year and the treatment was well tolerated. Only 15% patients had slight itching of the scalp for a few hours following injections. Most patients experienced tolerable pain while the injections were being administered.

The formulation consisting of (1) VEGF which is essential for angiogenesis and vascular permeability, may be responsible for maintaining proper vasculature around the hair follicle during the anagen growth phase, (2) Keratinocyte growth factor is highly very helpful in counteracting chemotherapy-induced alopecia, (3) Insulin-like growth factor 1 regulates cellular proliferation and migration and thus involved in promoting hair growth and it also prevents the follicle from entering catagen-like status, (4) Thymosin β4 promotes hair growth by influencing follicle stem cell growth, migration, differentiation, and protease production, (5) Basic FGF which promote hair growth by inducing the anagen phase in resting hair follicles, and (6) l-alanyl-l-histidyl–lysine-Cu^{2+} (AHK-Cu) copper tripeptide which promotes the growth of human hair follicles.

The author has compared this growth factors solution with PRP stating that in their procedure there is no need for blood collection, requirement of specialized equipment and standardization of procedure, effective dose calculation and duration of treatment.

Key Message

- *The growth factors cocktail if prepared in optimum concentration would be safe as well as efficacious in treating male and female pattern hair loss and alopecia, but requires further data for authentication.*

ARTICLE 89

Randomized Trial of Electrodynamic Microneedle Combined with 5% Minoxidil Topical Solution for the Treatment of Chinese Male Androgenetic Alopecia

Bao L, Gong L, Guo M, et al. Randomized trial of electrodynamic microneedle combined with 5% minoxidil topical solution for the treatment of Chinese male Androgenetic alopecia.
J Cosmet Laser Ther. 2017.

Abstract

Background: In treating androgenetic alopecia (AGA), 5% minoxidil is a commonly used topical drug. Using electrodynamic microneedle at the same time may increase absorption of minoxidil and further stimulate hair growth.

Objective: A 24-week, randomized, evaluator blinded, comparative study was performed to evaluate the efficacy of treating Chinese male AGA using microneedle combined with 5% minoxidil topical solution.

Methods: Randomized subjects received topical 5% minoxidil (group 1, n = 20), local electrodynamic microneedle treatments (group 2, n = 20) or local electrodynamic microneedle treatments plus topical 5% minoxidil (group 3, n = 20). A total of 12 microneedle treatments were performed every 2 weeks with 2 mL 5% minoxidil delivery in group 3 during each microneedle treatment. Patient receiving topical 5% minoxidil applied 1 mL of the solution twice daily over the course of the study. A total of 60 Chinese male subjects with Norwood-Hamilton type III–VI AGA were treated.

Results: The mean improvement in total hair density from baseline to 24 weeks was $18.8/cm^2$ in group 1, $23.4/cm^2$ in group 2 and $38.3/cm^2$ in group 3. The hair growth in the three groups was significantly different ($p = 0.002$), but there were no significant differences in toxicity found between the three groups.

Conclusion: Treatment with microneedle plus topical 5% minoxidil was associated with the best hair growth.

COMMENT

Treatments used to promote hair growth include 5α-reductase inhibitors, anti-androgenic drugs and topically applied minoxidil. Minoxidil is the only topical US Food and Drug Administration-approved drug for the treatment of androgenetic alopecia (AGA); other current medical treatments are often not successful and hair transplantation can be an expensive, painful procedure.

Minoxidil increases both the local blood supply with its direct vasodilator effects and the local expression of vascular endothelial growth factor (VEGF); together with these factors promotes angiogenesis of the dermal papilla.

Microneedling creates holes on the skin to damage the barrier of stratum corneum enabling easy entry of drugs into skin through microneedle holes and effects locally or enter into the capillary networks of dermis. Trauma seems to activate hair bulb stem cells, increasing the expression of VEGF and Wnt10b, which are genes associated with hair growth. Epidermal growth factors too get released during skin regeneration and repair. Use of microneedles could simulate this process.

An electrodynamic microneedle contains a disposable head with 9 needles that are 0.25 mm in diameter and have an adjustable length. When activated, the needles oscillate at a high frequency, diminishing needle pain and increasing drug delivery.

In treating AGA, using an electrodynamic microneedle may significantly improve the percutaneous absorption rate of minoxidil. The intense stimulation caused by microneedle at the local alopecia site may also give rise to hair follicle regrowth during the process of wound repair.

The best therapeutic effect was observed in cases treated with microneedle plus topical 5% minoxidil. The results were supported by the improvements seen in the nonvellus and the total hair counts, the hair thickness, investigator assessment and patient self-assessment. Patients of combination treatment had the best subjective cosmetic result.

Adverse events associated with the use of microneedle in treating AGA have not been previously reported; however, the use of microneedles may not be suitable in patients with altered immunity or cardiovascular disease because of the increase risk of infection and stress associated with the microneedle application. It is important to note that scalp infection and enlarged cervical lymph nodes were only seen in patients treated with microneedles.

Only two studies have reported the use of microneedles in treating male AGA. Dhurat R administered topical 5% minoxidil twice daily plus the application of microneedles once a week to treat 50 men with AGA while a control group received topical 5% minoxidil twice daily. The microneedle treatment group had the best outcome after 12 weeks of treatment.

The limitation in this study is the small number of patients to determine differences in their response rates, hair thickness, and the toxicity of different treatments. Further research should confirm the mechanisms of how microneedle treatments can promote hair growth or increase topical minoxidil absorption.

Key Messages

- *Microneedling enhances drug delivery through stratum corneum into dermis and dermal capillary network*
- *Trauma from microneedling stimulates hair regrowth by increasing VEGF and epidermal growth factors and Wnt10b gene expression pathway*
- *Combining topical minoxidil and electrodynamic microneedling offered better outcome in treatment of AGA than topical minoxidil or microneedling alone.*

ARTICLE 90

A Pilot Split-scalp Study of Combined Fractional Radiofrequency Microneedling and 5% Topical Minoxidil in Treating Male Pattern Hair Loss

Yu AJ, Luo YJ, Xu XG, et al. A pilot split-scalp study of combined fractional radiofrequency microneedling and 5% topical minoxidil in treating male pattern hair loss.
Clin Exp Dermatol. 2018;43(7):775-81.

Abstract

Various clinical trials have been conducted for management of male pattern hair loss (MPHL), but due to the limited outcome, there is a need for adjuvant therapies. Combined treatment with fractional radiofrequency microneedle (FRM) and 5% topical minoxidil could be an effective and safe adjuvant treatment option for MPHL in comparison with minoxidil alone.

COMMENT

Pattern hair loss (PHL), also called androgenetic alopecia (AGA), affects both men and women who are genetically predisposed. It is characterized by progressive nonscaring miniaturization of the hair follicle. It manifests as a gradual recession of the frontal hairline with thinning over parietal or vertex regions of the scalp.

Male PHL affects the quality of life and self-esteem of patients. Despite the high prevalence therapeutic options are limited. There are only two drugs approved by the Food and Drug Administration (FDA): (1) topical minoxidil and (2) oral finasteride. Due to poor compliance, there is a need for adjuvant therapy. There are many studies done on to stimulate the hair growth using energy-based devices like LLLT (low-level light therapy), erbium glass but with limited results. Hence there is a need to investigate different adjuvant therapies and procedures.

The study was done to know the efficacy and safety of combined FRM and 5% topical minoxidil in the treatment of MPHL. It was split scalp study where patient applied only minoxidil 5% tincture to one half of the scalp and other half was treated with radiofrequency microneedling five sessions at 4 weeks interval with minoxidil application. Phototrichogram and global assessment were done before and after 5 months of treatment. Assessment after 1 month of final session showed significant improvement in the combined therapy with respect to the hair count, hair thickness and photographic assessment. There were no adverse events noted.

Wounding stimulates hair follicle growth and regenerated hair follicles to establish a stem cell population. These stem cells have follicle differentiation with activation of the Wnt/beta-catenin pathway. The FRM device used produces both mechanical wounds by microneedles and thermal injury by radiofrequency. The FRM devise also reduce sebaceous activity by diminishing the sebaceous gland size and secretions. As AGA is associated with high oil secretions, the scalp and ensuring sebaceous secretions could add to the problems of AGA, AGA would be benefited by this mechanism of causing FRM by inflammation, which increases blood flow and follicular vascularization with increased delivery of minoxidil to the dermal papillae. Hence the combination treatment had shown both increase in hair count and hair thickness in comparison with minoxidil alone.

Key Message

- *MPHL is a very prevalent condition, the approved therapeutic options are limited. FRM plus minoxidil gave better results than minoxidil alone. FRM combined with topical minoxidil could be a novel treatment for MPHL, with good efficacy and minimal adverse events.*

ARTICLE 91

Combination of a Nonablative 1,927 nm Thulium Fiber Fractional Laser and Autologous Platelet-rich Plasma in Treatment of Male Androgenetic Alopecia: A Pilot Study

Brownell N, Panchaprateep R, Glinhom R. Combination of a non-ablative 1,927 nm thulium fiber fractional laser and autologous platelet-rich plasma in treatment of male androgenetic alopecia: A pilot study.
Chula Med J. 2019;63(1):13-21.

Abstract

Platelet-rich plasma (PRP) promotes hair growth by cell proliferation and prolonging anagen phase of hair follicles. Fractional laser might promote hair growth by creating proper wounding. This is a pilot study on nine men to investigate the efficacy and safety of the combination treatment of nonablative fractional laser and PRP in male androgenetic alopecia (AGA). Global photographs, trichoscan and patient self-assessment index were used to grade the results at the end of 6 months. There was increase in terminal hair density, total hair density and hair mass index with improvement in global photography. Adverse effects were transient erythema and mild burning sensation on the treated areas. The results of this small sample study can be considered safe and effective for the treatment of male AGA and create interest for further randomized, placebo-controlled trials.

COMMENT

Fractional laser therapy, autologous platelet-rich plasma (PRP), and hair transplantation are newer alternative modalities to treat androgenetic alopecia (AGA). The PRP is composed of multiple essential growth factors which stimulate hair growth by promoting cell proliferation, prolonging cell survival and the anagen phase of hair follicles. Fractional nonablative lasers either erbium/glass or thulium lasers with optimum settings have been found to stimulate hair growth by Wnt/beta-catenin pathway upregulation.

This trial aimed to investigate the efficacy and safety of a combination of nonablative fractional laser and PRP for the treatment of AGA as fractional laser could create proper wounding which resulted in subsequent platelet activation and might synergize with PRP in promoting hair proliferation. Fractional 1927 nm thulium-doped fiber laser with parameters of 3–5 Watts, 5–10 mJ/spot, 0.5–20 ms of pulse width, 3–5 passes followed by PRP injection was used on hair thinning area. Standardized global photographs assessment, targeted area hair mass index and patient self-assessment questionnaires were taken to evaluate hair growth.

Mean of platelets concentration in this study was 5.9 times higher compared to baseline which is considered a proper concentration. The results of the present study showed a significant increase in hair counts and hair density at both 3 months and 6 months after the last treatment. The adverse effects were mild and temporary as transient erythema and mild burning sensation over the treated area. The PRP injection was more painful compared to laser but within acceptable limits. Small sample size and lack of long-term follow-up were the drawbacks of the study.

Key Messages

- *Platelet-rich plasma is composed of multiple essential growth factors which stimulate hair growth by promoting cell proliferation, prolonging cell survival and the anagen phase of hair follicles*
- *Fractional nonablative lasers either erbium/glass or thulium lasers with optimum settings have been found to stimulate hair growth by Wnt/beta-catenin pathway upregulation*
- *Fractional laser could create proper wounding which resulted in subsequent platelet activation and might synergize with PRP in promoting hair proliferation*
- *Fractional CO_2 and erbium Yag can also be used along with PRP with minimum non-ablative parameters which are possible if proper understanding of lasers in hand.*

ARTICLE 92

Autologous Adipose Derived Stem Cell versus Platelet-rich Plasma Injection in the Treatment of Androgenetic Alopecia: Efficacy, Side Effects, and Safety

Kadry MH, El-Kheir WA, El-Sayed Shalaby M, et al. Autologous Adipose Derived Stem Cell versus Platelet Rich Plasma Injection in the Treatment of Androgentic Alopecia: Efficacy, Side Effects, and Safety.
J Clin Exp Dermatol Res. 2018;9:3.

Abstract

Background: Platelet-rich plasma (PRP) is based on the release of growth factors stimulating the initiation/extension of anagen phase as well as promoting vascularization. Adipose derived stem cell (AT-ADSCs) treatment was recently introduced as an alternative potential therapeutic application for hair growth.

Objective: The aim of this study was to assess the efficacy, side effects, and safety of AT-ADSCs and PRP in the treatment of androgenetic alopecia (AGA).

Patients and Methods: Sixty randomized patients were treated by PRP and AT-ADSCs. Each patient was evaluated and each lesion was treated by those modalities, patients received three sessions with 1 month interval for 3 months, follow-up after 3 months.

Results: A highly significant improvement <0.001 in terminal hair count of AT-ADSCs group as evaluated by videodermoscopy assessment of AGA; it was confirmed by highly significant improvement in intermediate hair count and mean caliber (<0.001), associated with high incidence of side effects especially headache and erythema. In contrast, PRP group showed significant improvement 0.037 in terminal hair count and non-significant improvement in intermediate hair count and mean caliber with minimum side effects. AT-ADSCs showed a significant improvement in terminal hair count than PRP, and highly significant improvement in intermediate hair count and hair caliber. Also, side effects of AT-ADSCs showed highly significant pain, headache and erythema but no serious adverse events.

Conclusion: Our study suggests that there was significant improvement in AGA after PRP and highly significant after AT-ADSCs therapy with significant difference of ADSC in terminal hair count and highly significant in caliber. Both modalities could effectively and safely be used to treat AGA.

COMMENT

Platelet-rich plasma (PRP) and AT-ADSCs are alternative potential therapeutic modalities for hair growth. This is a randomized, controlled, prospective single-blinded comparative clinical study to evaluate the efficacy, side effects, and safety of autologous ADSC versus PRP injection in the treatment of AGA. These adjuvant therapies (PRP and ADSCs) may help in stimulation and proliferation of stem cells, development of new follicles, and promoting neovascularization. The goal for treating alopecia with AT-ADSCs includes increasing the number of existing follicles.

Sixty patients older than 20 years, presenting with different grades of patterns of hair loss were eligible to participate in this 1 year study. The study patients did not use any other modalities of treatment for AGA during the course of the study. These patients were randomized in to two groups and subjected to the following treatment—AT-ADSCs and PRP.

They received three sessions with 1 month interval for 3 months and followed up after 3 months. Group 1 (30 patients) received PRP prepared with 8 mL of blood sample, centrifuged at 1,500 rpm for 5 minutes. The 0.1 mL intradermal (ID) injections were administered with 30 G needle spaced at 1 cm apart. In group 2 (30 patients) were treated by AT-ADSC and stromal vascular fraction (SVF). It was prepared from fat harvested by syringe aspiration with atraumatic cannula from the lower abdomen. After washing fat with sterile phosphate buffered saline (PBS), it was treated with 0.075% collagenase at 37°C for at least 30 minutes and later inactivated with Dulbecco's modified Eagle medium (DMEM). This was centrifuged at 1,200 × g (1,500 rpm) for 5 minutes. The SVF located in the pellet at the bottom of the lipoaspirate was collected in syringes and injected intradermal in the scalp. The patients were assessed by both videodermoscopic and photographic assessment. Videodermoscopic analysis assessed hair count including terminal hair (per square centimeter) and hair diameter. The photographic assessment included degree of improvement in grades and was assessed as mild and moderate improvement which implies that there is improvement within the same grade. It is considered good improvement if there is grade change, and, if the improvement causes change in the type to normal or type 1 then it is considered as an excellent improvement.

No significant difference between ADSC and PRP was noted in regard to medical and personal characteristics. In group 1, 46.66% (14 patients) on photographic assessment had no improvement. About 40% (12 patients) showed same grade mild photographic improvement. About 13.3% (4 patients) showed moderate photographic improvement in hair density and thickness but in same grade still.

In group 2, 30% (9 patients) on photographic improvement showed no improvement. About 30% (9 patients) showed same grade mild photographic improvement. About 26.6% (8 patients) showed moderate photographic improvement in hair density and thickness but still in the same grade. About 13.4% (14 patients) changed their grade from preceding grade and showed good improvement.

In PRP group, the mean terminal hair count changed from 68.87% ± 34.61 (before treatment) to 79.6% ± 38.27, after 3 months of last session of treatment and 10.73 ± 3.66 was the mean change of terminal hair density. Hair width increased 100 µm before treatment to 120 µm, 3 months after last session, showing significant progressive improvement. In the ADSC group, the mean terminal hair count before treatment was 58.3% ± 20.98% which increased after 3 months of last session of treatment to 77.6% ± 7.33%, and 19.30 ± 13.65 was the mean change of terminal hair density. Hair width increased 70 μm before treatment to 120 μm, 3 months after last session, showing significant progressive improvement. Pain, headache, and itching were the side effects in both the groups.

This is first clinical trial that compared PRP and ADSC in the treatment of AGA. PRP injections for hair restoration are minimally invasive and cost efficient treatment that increases hair density and diameter. ADSC are most promising stem cell population easily obtained in large quantities with little patient discomfort and considered as a promising therapy to promote hair growth via growth factor secretion.

There was significant improvement in AGA according to this study, after both PRP and after AT-ADSCs therapy (highly significant), with significant difference between both in terminal hair count and caliber (highly significant). Both modalities could safely and effectively be used in treatment of AGA. The significant long-term follow-up data was not done in this study, as subjects in majority were followed only for the 3 months in the treatment course.

Key Messages

- ADSCs injection being highly effective for alopecia, appears to be a new area of therapy under hair regeneration
- ADSC's injection increases hair diameter, hair density, and decreases the pull test to almost zero, thus promoting a good stability of the hair by increasing the hair density
- The treatment was not associated with any serious adverse events.

ARTICLE 93

Cellular Therapy with Human Autologous Adipose-derived Adult Cells of Stromal Vascular Fraction for Alopecia Areata

Anderi R, Nehman Makdissy N, Azar A, et al. Cellular therapy with human autologous adipose-derived adult cells of stromal vascular fraction for alopecia areata.
Stem Cell Res Ther. 2018 May 15;9(1):141.

Abstract

Background: Most common forms of hair loss (alopecia) are caused by aberrant hair follicle cycling and changes in hair follicle morphology. However, current treatments for alopecia do not specifically target these processes. Adipose-derived stromal vascular cells (ADSVCs) that can be harvested from fat cells are one of the latest breakthroughs in the aesthetic field. The potential use of stem cell-based therapies (SCBT) for the repair and regeneration of various tissues and organs offers a paradigm shift that may provide alternative therapeutic solutions, which can be applied to prevent hair loss. This study aimed to present clinical cases of SCBT for the treatment of alopecia areata by transplantation of ADSVCs in the scalp.

Methods: About 20 patients (9 women and 11 men) were recruited to our retrospectively registered study. After lipoaspiration, autologous ADSVCs were generated and characterized before the injection of 4–4.7×10^6 cells into the scalp of the patient. Hair regeneration was assessed by three clinical tests: the pull test, hair quality and hair density.

Results: All patients experienced hair regeneration, increased hair growth, and decreased pull test 3 and 6 months after the treatment with ADSVCs [hair density (85.1 ± 8.7 vs. 121.1 ± 12.5 hair/cm^2, $p < 0.0001$), hair diameter (60.5 ± 1.8 vs. 80.8 ± 2.4 µ, $p < 0.0001$) and pull-test values (4.4 ± 0.3 vs. 0.8 ± 0.2, $p < 0.0001$), untreated versus 6 months postoperative. Significant variation was observed between men and women only for hair diameter. No significant differences were observed with age.

Conclusion: The obtained results prove the efficacy and the safety of the treatment, and satisfaction of the patients confirms the quality of the results.

COMMENT

Multipotent stem cells within adipose tissue, existing in adipose-derived stromal vascular cells (ADSVCs), are a promising stem cell population for follicular remodeling. In present study, efficacy of autologous ADSVCs graft in alopecia areata is studied and also the safety and effectiveness of the transplantation. ADSVCs release growth factors, promotes increased neovascularization and hair regeneration. The clinical trial included 20 white healthy subjects (n = 20, 38.3 ± 2.3 years, 9 women and 11 men) from the Middle East.

ADSVC preparation and treatment protocol: Abdominal fat lipoaspirate was collected and diluted with sterile phosphate buffered saline (PBS), Sigma-Aldrich (St. Louis, MO, USA) and antibiotics; centrifuged at $430 \times g$ for 10 minutes (without brakes). The wash step done 2–3 times and later floating adipose tissue was digested with an equal volume of collagenase type 1 [10 mg/mL in PBS containing 5 mM Ca^{2+}/Mg^{2+} (C0130, Sigma-Aldrich), final concentration of 0.5%] at 37°C for 30 minutes with shaking (250 rpm). The collagenase was inactivated and the sample was centrifuged at $600 \times g$ for 10 minutes. Cell pellet obtained was resuspended in NaCl 0.9% and filtered through a 100 µm cell strainer to remove debris. After centrifugation (300 RCF/5 min), 5 mL of the stromal vascular fraction was collected. All the processing must be realized within a maximal time of 90 minutes. The number of viable cells were determined manually (trypan blue method) and validated on MACSQuant analyzer (7AAD staining method). Processing of all samples was done within 120 minutes and transplanted within 3 hours. Immunophenotyping of freshly isolated ADSVCs was also done by flow cytometry; cell viability was assessed using the trypan blue exclusion assay, and validated by 7AAD method by flow cytometry. The telomerase activity was assessed by real-time qPCR using the Quantitative Telomerase Detection Kit.

Adipose-derived stromal vascular cells were injected into the scalp; 5 mL was injected in 25 spots; 0.2 mL per injection delivered perpendicularly, separated by 1 cm in a square shape all over the scalp, depth attained 4 mm. The 0.2 mL containing $0.160–0.188 \times 10^6$ cells were injected per spot; total number of $4–4.7 \times 10^6$ cells were transplanted; 4×10^6 total cells/25 spots/per subject = minimum concentration of 160,000 cells/spot of injection. This maintained the minimum levels of CD105+ and CD166+ cells per injection and avoided any aggregation of the cells. Follow-up was performed at 1 week, 3 months and 6 months.

About 19 out of 20 patients showed improved hair diameter. Hair pull test showed a significant decrease in the number of extracted hair (p <0.0001); 0.80 ± 0.17 and 0.90 ± 0.20 versus 4.35 ± 0.33 for 6 and 3 months postoperatively versus baseline. Hair diameter increased significantly (p <0.0001) especially after 6 months; 80.8 ± 2.4 μ and 62.8 ± 1.7 μ versus 60.5 ± 1.8 μ for 6 and 3 months postoperatively vs. baseline. Hair density was also significantly (p <0.0001) augmented; 121.1 ± 12.5 and 120.8 ± 12.6 versus 85.1 ± 8.7 for 6 and 3 months postoperatively versus baseline. The mean growth was approximately 36%, and the optimal effect was 61.2%.

Transplantation of autologous ADSVCs was found to be safe, effective, and an encouraging cell-based therapy for the treatment of alopecia and as a nonsurgical hair loss treatment. The efficacy of ADSVCs in grade III and advanced cases of alopecia areata needs to be established. In the study, ADSVCs have been tried in untreated cases, whereas their role in conventional treatment resistant alopecia areata also needs to be looked into.

Key Messages

- Adipose-derived stromal vascular cells for the treatment of alopecia have shown promising results similar to hematopoietically derived plasma or ADSVC conditioned medium (ADSVC-CM)
- This research article has a lot of technical evaluation done by authors, but the definition of cases with respect to alopecia types is varied. There is no clarity on alopecia types. The tittle says it is done for alopecia areata but the selection also includes patterned hair loss patients. The study does not show global photographs of treated cases.

ARTICLE 94

Conventional and Novel Stem Cell-based Therapies for Androgenic Alopecia

Talavera-Adame D, Newman D, Newman N. Conventional and novel stem cell-based therapies for androgenic alopecia. *Stem Cells Cloning.* 2017;10:11-19.

Abstract

The prevalence of androgenetic alopecia (AGA) increases with age and it affects both men and women. Patients diagnosed with AGA may experience decreased quality of life, depression and feel self-conscious. There are a variety of therapeutic options ranging from prescription drugs to nonprescription medications. Currently, AGA involves an annual global market revenue of US$4 billion and a growth rate of 1.8%, indicating a growing consumer market. Although natural and synthetic ingredients can promote hair growth and, therefore, be useful to treat AGA; some of them have important adverse effects and unknown mechanisms of action that limit their use and benefits. Biologic factors that include signaling from stem cells (SCs), dermal papilla cells (DPCs), and platelet-rich plasma (PRP) are some of the current therapeutic agents being studied for hair restoration with milder side effects. However, most of the mechanisms exerted by these factors in hair restoration are still being researched. In this review, we analyze the therapeutic agents that have been used for AGA and emphasize the potential of new therapies based on advances in SC technologies and regenerative medicine.

COMMENT

Androgenetic alopecia (AGA) prevalence increases with age and it affects both women and men. One of the targets for stem cell (SC) technologies is hair restoration, to restore the hair in AGA. To promote hair regrowth, several SC factors such as peptides exert essential signals. The differentiation of SCs to keratinocytes occurs by stimulation of some of these signals which are important for hair follicle (HF) growth. Other signals can promote SC proliferation in the HF by stimulation of dermal papilla cells (DPCs). The author here aims to describe characteristics of HFs and discuss different treatment modality used for AGA currently and possible hair regeneration novel agents.

Hair follicle stem cells (HFSCs) are located in the bulge region of the HF and they have interaction with the dermal papillary mesenchymal SCs (MSCs). They promote activation of few cellular pathways essential for DPC function, growth and survival, like the Wnt signaling pathway activation. Other signals which are essential for HF maintenance are those from endothelial cells (ECs) at the dermal papilla. HFSCs undergo a short proliferative phase in which they produce new hair and self-renew, during early anagen stage. Therefore, bulge region has a SC niche that makes multiple signals toward proliferation or quiescence stages. An important role in maintaining the threshold for HFSC activation is by Forkhead box C1 (FOXC1) transcription factor. The knock down of these in the bulge area cells reduces the threshold for proliferation of the cells, and the anagen cycle starts with increased frequency due to shorter periods of time taken for promotion of HFSC proliferation. The drugs and treatment modalities for AGA are—Minoxidil, finasteride, dutasteride, latanoprost/bimatoprost, low level laser therapy (LLLT), Apple Procyanidin B-2, Procerin, Provillus, Follicusan, Musol 20, Capixyl, Tricholastyl, EMortal Pep, Planoxia-RG, Keramino-25, Seveov, HairOmega, green tea, Nioxin, alfatradiol and quercetin.

The HF is a complex structure that grows when adequate signaling is provided to the HFSCs. SCs in culture promote hair growth by activation of HFSCs and DPCs. The study of these signals can allow to gain the necessary knowledge for developing more effective treatment modality in the management of AGA with minimal adverse effects. Novel therapeutic options may be generated by further studies in the field of regenerative medicine.

There is a lot of research going into SC therapy for hair disorders. Some centers are also trying tissue micrografts containing various SC population from all components of skin and subcutaneous tissue. The progress made in this field is quite significant so far extrapolation to clinical efficacy is awaited.

> **Key Messages**
> - The HF is a complex structure that grows when adequate signaling is provided to the HFSCs
> - Stem cells in culture are able to activate DPCs and HFSCs and, subsequently promote hair growth.

ARTICLE 95

Systemic Photodynamic Therapy in Folliculitis Decalvans

Collier NJ, Allan D, Diaz Pesantes F, et al. Systemic photodynamic therapy in folliculitis decalvans.
Clin Exp Dermatol. 2018;43(1):46-9.

Abstract

Folliculitis decalvans (FD) is a neutrophilic cicatricial alopecia due to dysfunctional immune activity. The role of *Staphyloccoccus aureus* is presumed to be vital. Treatment includes antibiotics and anti-inflammatory agents. Topical photodynamic therapy (PDT) has also been used. The authors have successfully treated a patient of FD with systemic PDT, which was nonresponsive to commonly used topical and systemic therapies.

COMMENT

Folliculitis decalvans presents with recurrent episodes of pustules, healing with cicatricial alopecia. As the etiology is immune dysfunction and *Staphyloccoccus aureus* infection, the treatment options are antibiotics like doxycycline, rifampicin and clindamycin, retinoids (isotretinoin and acitretin), prednisolone and ciclosporin. In this report, as the patient had not responded to the above therapies, authors have administered systemic photodynamic therapy (PDT) using ultraviolet light (100–140 J/cm^2) with porfimer sodium 1 mg/kg as monotherapy. Porfimer sodium 1 mg/kg was administered as a slow intravenous injection (porfimer sodium 75 mg powder reconstituted in 31.8 mL 5% glucose solution), then 48 hours later the clinically affected scalp skin was treated by illumination with 630 nm red light.

Systemic PDT with porfimer sodium is substantially more effective than 5-aminolevulinic acid in killing *S. aureus* in vitro. Systemic PDT causes local immunomodulation, and thus improved scar healing. There is no risk of resistance, unlike antibiotics. Also, systemic PDT allows more photosensitizing drugs to be delivered to deep dermis and subcutaneous fat, unlike topical therapy. As porfimer sodium has a long half-life of 17 days, photoprotection of eyes and skin should be recommended for 30 days postprocedure. No major side effects were noted in this patient. One more advantage of this therapy is improvement in scarring which is otherwise not noted with systemic antibiotic therapy.

Key Messages

- *Systemic photodynamic therapy is an option when other modes like antibiotics and anti-inflammatory agents have failed in treatment of FD.*
- *Porfimer sodium appears to be better efficacious than 5ALA.*

Section 5 Diagnostic and Investigative Trichology

ARTICLE 96

Nanotechnology Advances for Hair Loss

Pereira MN, Ushirobira CY, Cunha-Filho MS, et al. Nanotechnology advances for hair loss. *Ther Deliv. 2018;9(8):593-603.*

Abstract

Alopecia is progressive hair loss from scalp or any other body's region. Androgenetic alopecia (AGA) and alopecia areata (AA) are the most common types of alopecia affecting both men and women. Most of the approved treatments have no definitive therapeutic regimen and have serious adverse effects. This article highlights the nanoencapsulation improving the therapeutic outcome of this pathology, promoting a targeted drug delivery with enhanced local bioavailability which could reduce the adverse effects.

COMMENT

Androgenetic alopecia (AGA) and alopecia areata (AA), the most common types of alopecia, affect both men and women with minor cosmetic issue but causing major psychological distress leading to anxiety and depression. It affects around 50% of men between 30 and 50 years and 15–30% of women in their 30s. In AGA, the Food and Drug Administration approved treatments are 2% and 5% minoxidil solution and foam twice daily. Oral finasteride (1 mg/day) is only approved for men. Adverse events with these medications lead to the poor compliance leading to advent of newer technology called nanotechnology with targeted drug delivery with less adverse events.

Nanosystems are composed of lipids in solid state or a solid matrix trapping a mixture of liquid, amorphous or unsaturated lipids (nanostructured lipid carrier). Other nanosystems include liposomes, ethosomes, niosomes, lipid nanoparticles and polymeric nanoparticles. Nanosystem control drug release, proportionating equal effect with fewer administrations and solving irritation problems related to the formulation.

Solid lipid nanoparticles have presented good permeation results, but stability became a constant issue as solid lipids may form crystalline networks, leading to drug expulsion during storage. To overcome this, nanostructured lipid carrier was introduced, an oil-based nanoparticle containing a solid unstructured lipid core that allows the encapsulation of lipophilic drugs with increased entrapment efficiency and drug retention during storage.

Liposomes, consisting mainly of phospholipids, are spherical vesicular structures comprising a two-layer membrane as a hydrophobic compartment and an aqueous core. Lipophilic nature of the liposomes makes it an effective agent for penetrating the lipid-filled hair follicles. Thereby, it increases the ease of penetration and absorption of active ingredients. Transfersomes include edge activators in their composition, providing higher vesicle flexibility for easy penetration. Niosomes are nonionic surfactant-based vesicles with high stability, biodegradable and biocompatible compositions. Niosomes encapsulate various lipophilic and hydrophilic drugs, proteins and genes. Main disadvantages associated with liposomes such as high cost and purity problems commonly associated with phospholipids. The polymeric nanoparticles have the ability to protect encapsulated drugs from degradation, increasing shelf life of the drug.

Nanoparticulated systems are also presented as an alternative to oral administration. Eudragit E nanoparticle containing dutasteride showed a better drug absorption in rats, with an expressive increase in bioavailability compared with dutasteride suspension. Also finasteride nanosuspensions showed higher bioavailability parameters than pure drug or even microparticles.

Key Messages
- Nanosystems promote a superior drug accumulation in the skin in relation to conventional non-particulate systems. Nanosystems such as liposomes, ethosomes, niosomes, lipid nanoparticles and polymeric nanoparticles are being investigated for follicular targeting drug delivery
- Nanoparticles with smaller diameters tend to penetrate deeper into the hair follicles, settling into the hair bulb
- Follicular accumulation of the lipidic nanosystems occurs through an interaction of the lipids composing the nanosystem with the sebum present in the cutaneous appendix.

ARTICLE 97

Parietal Scalp is Another Affected Area in Female Pattern Hair Loss: An Analysis of Hair Density and Hair Diameter

Rojhirunsakool S, Suchonwanit P. Parietal scalp is another affected area in female pattern hair loss: an analysis of hair density and hair diameter.
Clin Cosmet Investig Dermatol. 2017;11:7-12.

Abstract
This study aimed to correlate the quantitative measurement with the clinical presentation of female pattern hair loss (FPHL) by investigating normal women and FPHL patients. Total 471 FPHL

patients and 236 normal women were investigated to know the characteristics of hair density and hair diameter; various areas of the scalp were assessed by using a computerized handheld USB camera. In normal women highest hair density was in mid scalp and lowest in parietal region, whereas the lowest hair density was seen in the parietal area in FPHL group. The study throws insight on the parietal area, another affected area in FPHL in addition to the mid scalp area.

COMMENT

In this study, automated phototrichogram was used which combines the use of a digital video microscope with an image analysis system for measurement of hair dynamics. In this study, apart from measuring the hair density and hair diameter of scalp hair in normal women and female pattern hair loss (FPHL) patients, there is an analysis on the correlation between the quantitative measurements obtained by computer-assisted software compared with the clinical presentation of FPHL.

All four areas, mid scalp, frontal, occipital and parietal areas were evaluated. The hair density, diameter of nonvellus hair and the percentage of miniaturized hair were performed using a computerized handheld USB camera with computer-assisted software. Digital images were recorded in 50-fold magnification.

There was an increase in miniaturized hair on the parietal area of patients with FPHL which has never been described before. Because frontal and parietal scalps share their embryological background, i.e. neural crest, the pathophysiology of parietal scalp involvement in FPHL could be explained by increased 5α-reductase enzyme in this area compared to unaffected scalp. All parameters (hair density, nonvellus hair diameter and percentage of miniaturized hair) were correlated well with clinical Ludwig staging. However, hair density and percentage of miniaturized hair were more consistent and sensitive than nonvellus hair diameter.

Key Messages

- The measurement of hair density and diameter by computer-assisted software offers practitioners quantitative data to identify the FPHL
- Parietal area is also significantly affected in FPHL with reduced hair density and percentage of miniaturized hair follicles
- The recently described entity called DUPA, diffuse unpatterned hair loss, is more commonly seen in female patients. Studies have to be conducted with regard to early involvement of parietal scalp to predict onset of DUPA in females
- In hair transplantation among female patients, the surgeons need to keep in mind the involvement of parietal scalp while choosing donor area.

ARTICLE 98

"Normal-appearing" Scalp Areas are also Affected in Lichen Planopilaris and Frontal Fibrosing Alopecia: An Observational Histopathologic Study of 40 Patients

Doche I, Romiti R, Hordinsky MK, et al. "Normal-appearing" scalp areas are also affected in lichen planopilaris and frontal fibrosing alopecia: An observational histopathologic study of 40 patients.
Exp Dermatol. 2018;7.

Abstract

This is an observational histopathologic study of 40 patients of lichen planopilaris (LPP) or frontal fibrosing alopecia (FFA), who were evaluated for histopathologic changes in affected and unaffected scalp and were compared with histologic features of healthy control subjects and also with clinical signs and scalp symptoms. The normal appearing scalp without clinical lesions also showed lymphocytic perifollicular inflammation around the isthmus/infundibulum in 65% of cases, perifollicular fibrosis in 15% and mucin deposits in 7.5% of the cases. There was no direct correlation between the degree of histopathological inflammation, and scalp symptoms and clinical lesions. This study insights that both diseases might have generalized processes on scalp and therefore, need systemic or complete topical scalp therapy.

COMMENT

Lichen planopilaris (LPP) and frontal fibrosing alopecia (FFA) are primary lymphocytic cicatricial alopecia, affecting the area of follicular stem cells. It is known that these disorders show involvement of the hair follicular infundibulum and isthmus in the affected area of the scalp. This study is based on the presence of histopathological features of LPP and FFA, in clinically normal appearing scalp. The authors claim that this is a pioneer study.

This hospital-based, case-control study was conducted at the University of Sao Paulo, Brazil. About 40 patients with LPP in 12, and FFP in 28, along with these 11 healthy controls were included in this study. The patients and the controls underwent two 4 mm punch scalp biopsies, in patients of cicatricial alopecia they were taken from the most affected and nonaffected scalp, whereas in healthy controls they were taken from the similar matched areas. Lichen Planopilaris Activity Index (LPPAI) was used for clinical assessment. The clinical features like diffuse erythema, perifollicular erythema and perifollicular scaling were assessed in affected scalp. Unaffected scalp was classified based on normal hair density, null LPPAI scoring, and unremarkable clinical findings. The histopathological evaluation was done for the vertical sections obtained, after hematoxylin and eosin staining, and assessed for perifollicular inflammation, perifollicular fibrosis, and mucin deposits. Out of 40 patients enrolled in the study, 65% showed perifollicular lymphocytic infiltrate in unaffected scalp. Perifollicular fibrosis and perifollicular mucin deposition were also seen in LPP and FFA group.

The assessment of only vertical sections and performing only qualitative assessment, and not quantitative assessment by dermatopathologist limits this study.

The autoimmune disorders, LPP and FFA, most commonly affect only certain areas of the scalp. The diagnosis of both the disorders depends on both clinical and histopathological features. Though both the disorders have almost similar features, they differ in their progression with LPP having fast and devasting progression and FFA developing slowly. The occurrence of histopathological features in normal looking scalp suggests that only certain areas of the scalp are prone to cicatricial alopecia. This study also validates the need for total scalp treatment and also usage of systemic medicines to prevent progression. This study urges the hair biologist to extend their research to involve both affected and normal looking scalp.

Key Messages

- The inflammatory diseases like LPP and FFA are likely to involve the entire scalp progressively. The initial observation of FFA involving only frontal scalp is modified as disease was observed in occipital as well as back of the scalp
- The cicatricial alopecia, LPP and FFA are more generalized processes involving whole scalp, with certain areas more prone to develop clinical manifestations
- Total scalp therapy and systemic medications should be started on diagnosis to prevent further progression of the disease process
- The therapeutic response to systemic agents like cyclosporine in LPP and dihydrotestosterone inhibitors in FFA also points toward slow involvement of the entire scalp in both these disorders.

ARTICLE 99

First Order Derivative Spectrophotometric Method for Determination of Minoxidil and Finasteride in Pharmaceutical Dosage Form

Aishwarya R, Madhuri H, Shuchi D. First order derivative spectrophotometric method for determination of minoxidil and finasteride in pharmaceutical dosage form.
J Pharm Sci Bioscientific Res. 2018;8(1):112-6.

Abstract

This article highlights on use of a simple and precise first-order derivative spectrophotometric method for validation of minoxidil (MXD) and finasteride (FIN) in pharmaceutical dose. The linearity for MXD and FIN was obtained in the concentration range 5–25 µg/mL and 0.1–0.5 µg/mL with 0.9990 and 0.9971 correlation coefficient, respectively; with methanol and water, the quantitative determination was carried out using first-order spectra of MIN at 300 nm [zero crossing point (ZCP) of FIN] and FIN at 228.63 nm (ZCP of MIN).

COMMENT

Minoxidil (MXD), chemically known as 6-(Piperidin-1-yl) pyrimidine-2, 4-diamine 3-oxide, is an antihypertensive agent used in the treatment of male pattern hair loss. It acts by prolonging anagen stage by its anti-apoptotic effect on dermal papillary cells. FIN, chemically known as N-(1,1-dimethylethyl)-3-oxo-(5α, 17β)-4-azaandrost-1-ene-17-carboxamide, belongs to the class anti-androgen, an oral agent which is a 5-α reductase inhibitor. Literature survey has used second-order derivative spectroscopy and reverse phase high performance liquid chromatography (RP-HPLC) analytical methods for MXD and FIN in combined dosage form. This article involves validation of simple, precise, sensitive and accurate first-order ultraviolet (UV) spectrophotometric method for estimation of MXD and FIN in pharmaceutical dosage form according to ICH guideline.

In the study, double beam UV-visible spectrophotometer having two matched quartz cells with 1 cm light path and single pan electronic analytical balance (REPTECH) was used. Pure form of MXD and FIN with methanol and water as solvent was chosen. Zero crossing point (ZCP) value of MXD was found to be 300 nm for estimation of FIN and ZCP value of FIN was found to be 228.63 nm for estimation of MXD because adequate absorbance is produced at this wavelength. The validation parameter assessed included linearity, precision, assay procedure, limit of detection and limit of quantification. Recovery study was carried out showing accuracy with % recovery of 98.93–99.95% for MXD and 99.61–99.82% for FIN. Pharmaceutical dosage form was analyzed by the developed method and the assay was found to be 99.19% and 99.53% for MXD and FIN, respectively.

Key Message

- *First-order derivative UV spectroscopic method has been found simple, accurate and precise method for estimation of pharmaceutical dosage form of MXD and FIN.*

ARTICLE 100

Salivary Sex Hormones in Adolescent Females with Trichotillomania

Grant JE, Chamberlain SR. Salivary sex hormones in adolescent females with trichotillomania.
Psychiatry Res. 2018;265:221-3.

Abstract

Trichotillomania is several times more common in women and has peak onset around puberty. The role of sex hormones, however, has received little research. About 11 adolescent girls with trichotillomania, postmenarche and not taking birth control, were examined on a variety of clinical measures. Participants provided saliva samples for analysis of estradiol, progesterone and testosterone levels. Lower progesterone was associated with more severe symptoms and lower levels of all hormones were associated with worse overall functioning. Adolescents with trichotillomania exhibit a range of hormone levels but that lower levels of certain hormones may have important clinical associations.

COMMENT

This article is based on the concept of increased incidence of trichotillomania in adolescent females. The authors have tried to find a correlation of salivary sex hormones levels in adolescent female patients with trichotillomania.

This study included 11 adolescent girls with prior diagnosis of trichotillomania, who had attained menarche. The saliva sample was obtained and stored at −20°C. The study participants were assessed for the levels of estradiol, progesterone and testosterone in their salivary samples. This was done with the standard radioimmunological methodology. The severity of trichotillomania, psychosocial dysfunction and quality of life was assessed using Massachusetts General Hospital Hair Pulling Scale, NIMH Trichotillomania Severity Scale (NIMH-TSS) and Sheehan Disability scale (SDS).

On assessment, the patients showed moderate symptom severity of trichotillomania based on NIMH-TSS scale. Overall, the patients had lower progesterone levels, and lower levels of all the three hormones were associated with worst prognosis, which was assessed using SDS scale.

Progesterone, through its metabolite allopregnanolone, acts on GABA receptor, and has a role on adaptive response to stress. The association of lower levels of hormones with higher disability implicates dysregulation of these hormones in pathophysiology of trichotillomania, which merits further studies.

The point which limits this study is the sample size, which is very small, hence cannot be generalized to wider population. The psychometric properties of the clinical scales could not be assessed in this study due to small sample size. There was no matched control group in this study for comparison. Other hormones like luteinizing hormone, follicle-stimulating hormone and gonadotropin-releasing hormone were not examined. Finally, the most important one is that the values obtained were not reported in conjunction with menstrual cycle.

The hormonal changes seen in the adolescent trichotillomania patients, if done as larger studies, would open doors for new therapeutic modalities. Lower levels of these hormones in trichotillomania patients validate the need for further interventions.

> **Key Messages**
> - Lower levels of key sex hormones (progesterone, estradiol, and testosterone) are associated with higher disability in adolescent females with trichotillomania. The study particularly points toward progesterone involvement in trichotillomania and further studies by therapy intervention with progestin supplements would be in a place in due course of time
> - The need for future studies on salivary sex hormones in trichotillomania, and validating these to suggest new therapeutic directions.

ARTICLE 101

Inflammasome Activation Characterizes Lesional Skin of Folliculitis Decalvans

Eyraud A, Milpied B, Thiolat D, et al. Inflammasome activation characterizes lesional skin of folliculitis decalvans. *Acta Derm Venereol. 2018;98(6):570-5.*

Abstract

Folliculitis decalvans (FD) is a chronic disease of inflammatory origin, with poorly defined pathogenesis, leading to scarring alopecia. The aim of this study was to investigate the expression of interleukin (IL)-1β and IL-8, inflammasome (NALP1 and NALP3), and type I interferon (MxA), the markers associated with the activation of innate immune signals. This is a retrospective monocentric study, it included 17 patients of biopsy-proven FD. Disease activity (active vs. stable) was defined histologically and clinically. Immunostaining was done using antibodies directed against IL-1β, IL-8, NALP1, NALP3 and MxA on skin biopsies of FD. Results were compared with lichen planopilaris (LPP) and normal controls. Six patients had stable disease and 11 had active disease. IL-1β, NALP1 and NALP3 expression were significantly higher in hair follicles in FD compared with LPP and controls. This study concludes that, in FD, inflammasome activation is associated predominantly with immune system, suggesting the role of IL-1β blockade in FD.

COMMENT

Folliculitis decalvans (FD) is a long-standing chronic inflammatory disease which leads to primary cicatricial alopecia. The FD is characterized by occurrence of patches of alopecia, predominantly in vertex and occipital area, associated with recurrent perifollicular erythema, follicular pustules and hemorrhagic crusts. It is characterized by perifollicular neutrophilic infiltrate involving the upper and middle part of the follicle.

The pathogenesis of FD has been uncertain. The role of microbiota dysbiosis and inflammatory pathway has been implicated. The presence of inflammasomes is already known in neutrophil-rich dermatitis. This study analyzed innate immunity, by the presence and intensity of markers associated with inflammasome: NALP1, NALP3, IL-1β and IL-8 which leads to the recruitment of neutrophils.

In this case-control study, 17 patients of stable and active FD were evaluated, along with patients with lichen planopilaris (LPP) and healthy controls. The skin biopsy samples obtained were assessed by immunohistochemistry using semi-quantitative methods for NALP1, NALP3, IL-1β and MxA. The epidermal expression of these components was same in both FD and LPP, however, there was higher follicular expression of NALP1 and NALP3 in FD as compared to LPP, and there was higher expression of IL-8 in the dermis of FD whereas LPP and controls showed no to minimal expression. FD patients did not show the presence of type 1 interferon as seen in LPP.

This study showed that there is no difference between active and stable FD, implying that there is persistent inflammation due to bacterial biofilms in stable LPP. The role of inflammasomes activation has been considered in pathogenesis of FD, this opens new horizons with respect to therapeutic modalities for FD and supports the view of usage of IL-1β blockade therapy in its management.

Key Messages

- *Folliculitis decalvans is characterized by increased expression of inflammasomes: NALP1, NALP3 and IL-1β*
- *There is no difference between active and stable forms of FD*
- *Folliculitis decalvans is one of the most challenging conditions to be treated and IL-1β blockade therapy can help to improve its management*
- *IL-1β blocking drugs like etanercept, infliximab and anakinra theoretically can be used. Adalimumab is the recent biologic which has been tried in FD in stray reports.*

ARTICLE 102

Ultraviolet Filters in Hair-care Products: A Possible Link with Frontal Fibrosing Alopecia and Lichen Planopilaris

Callander J, Frost J, Stone N. Ultraviolet filters in hair-care products: a possible link with frontal fibrosing alopecia and lichen planopilaris.
Clin Exp Dermatol. 2018;43(1):69-70.

Abstract

Frontal fibrosing alopecia (FFA) and lichen planopilaris (LPP) are autoimmune, primary lymphocytic cicatricial alopecia. Environmental factors are known to trigger these conditions in predisposed individuals. This study highlights that ultraviolet (UV) filters used in hair-care products are possible trigger in initiation or progression of the disease.

COMMENT

Ultraviolet (UV) filters are traditionally known to be present in facial cosmetic products. The use of sunscreens and facial products have increased in the recent times, which would explain the increased incidence of frontal fibrosing alopecia (FFA) in the past decade, and also the occurrence of FFA besides facial skin over the hair margin. The author highlights that UV filters are also present in hair-care products to prevent photodegradation during storage. They are added in color-protect type products, leave-on-products to protect the hair from UV damage, and in shampoos and conditioners. This forms the basis of involvement of wider area of the scalp in FFA and lichen planopilaris (LPP). According to this article, cent percent of the patients with either FFA or LPP were using wash out hair-care products and 91% of them using leave-in hair-care products.

The knowledge of hair-care products and sunscreens with UV filters would help the dermatologists to control the trigger and also provide basis of progressive pattern of FFA and LPP.

Key Messages
- Awareness about frequent use of sunscreen chemicals in both leave-in and wash-off hair-care products
- Sunscreen chemicals may play a role in development of FFA and LPP, the fact is yet to be validated by large clinical studies.

ARTICLE 103

Staphylococcus aureus is the Most Common Bacterial Agent of the Skin Flora of Patients with Seborrheic Dermatitis

Tamer F, Yuksel ME, Sarifakioglu E, et al. Staphylococcus aureus is the most common bacterial agent of the skin flora of patients with seborrheic dermatitis.
Dermatol Pract Concept. 2018;8(2):80–84.

Abstract

Background: Seborrheic dermatitis is an inflammatory skin disease that affects 1–3% of the general population. The *Malassezia* species has been implicated as the main causative agent; however, the bacterial flora of the skin may also play role in the etiopathogenesis. Therefore, we investigated the most common bacterial agent of the skin flora of patients with seborrheic dermatitis.

Materials and Methods: About 51 patients with seborrheic dermatitis and 50 healthy individuals were included in this study. Sterile cotton swabs were rubbed on the scalp of the participants for bacterial culture. Colonial morphology was identified with gram stain and catalase test.

Results: *Staphylococcus aureus* was isolated from 25 (49%) patients with seborrheic dermatitis and 10 (20%) healthy individuals within the control group. Coagulase-negative staphylococci were isolated from 24 (47.1%) patients with seborrheic dermatitis and 17 (34%) healthy individuals within the control group. Diphtheroids were present in 2 (3.9%) patients and 1 (2%) subject within the control group. Gram-negative bacilli were present only in 1 (2%) patient. Hemolytic streptococci and bacilli were identified in 1 (2%) subject from each group. Colonization of coagulase-negative staphylococci, diphtheroids, gram-negative bacilli, hemolytic streptococci, and bacillus did not differ between patients and healthy controls. However, *S. aureus* colonization was significantly more common in patients with seborrheic dermatitis than in healthy controls.

Conclusion: Within this study, we revealed that *S. aureus* colonization was significantly higher among the patients. Therefore, we propose that, in addition to the *Malassezia* species, *S. aureus* may play a role in the etiopathogenesis of seborrheic dermatitis.

COMMENT

The etiopathogenesis of seborrheic dermatitis is not clearly understood and *Malassezia* species has been implicated as the main causative agent. In addition, few studies were for and against of Demodex mite in causing seborrheic dermatitis. There have been a few studies investigating the bacterial flora of the patients with seborrheic dermatitis.

This study reveals that *Staphylococcus aureus* and coagulase-negative *Staphylococcus* were the most common bacteria isolated from the patient and control groups, respectively.

Also *S. aureus* was significantly more frequent in the skin lesions of patients with seborrheic dermatitis (49%) than in healthy subjects within the control group (20%) followed by coagulase-negative *Staphylococcus* in patients (47.1%) than in healthy subjects (34%).

The authors conclude bacterial diversity in the skin lesions of seborrheic dermatitis as interactions between *Malassezia* species and bacterial flora of the skin seem to be associated with the development of seborrheic dermatitis. They propose *S. aureus* may play a role. Therefore, appropriate antibiotic therapy should be considered in the treatment of severe and persistent seborrheic dermatitis cases.

Key Messages

- *Staphylococcus aureus may play significant role in development of seborrheic dermatitis by interacting with Malassezia species*
- *It is to be noted that patients with seborrheic dermatitis of scalp are also known to develop seborrheic folliculitis which is more common when compared to normal population. Many a times, cultures appear to be negative. This study brings out facts on colonization of Staphylococcus in normal patients and seborrheic dermatitis patients, it shows colonization is increased by more than two times in seborrheic dermatitis patients. This probably indicates S. aureus as a contributor to pathogenesis rather than bystander*
- *Appropriate antibiotic therapy can help in treatment of severe and persistent seborrheic dermatitis cases and may also prevent recurrences.*

ARTICLE 104

Assessment of Heavy Metal and Trace Element Levels in Patients with Telogen Effluvium

Yavuz IH, Yavuz GO, Bilgili SG, et al. Assessment of heavy metal and trace element levels in patients with telogen effluvium.
Indian J Dermatol. 2018;63(3):246-50.

Abstract

Background: Despite a multitude of literature, etiology of primary chronic telogen effluvium (TE) remains incompletely known. Essential heavy metals are known to have beneficial effects in living organisms including humans. However, when the higher tolerable limits are exceeded, they may lead to toxic effects. The aim of this study is to assess the levels of heavy metals and trace elements in patients with chronic TE.

Materials and Methods: A total of 40 patients with chronic TE were included in this study, and 30 healthy women were considered as control. Dermatological and general examination was done in all individuals. Trichogram was done in patients with positive hair pull test. Trichogram showing the presence of >20% telogen hair was a requirement for the inclusion in the study. Serum trace element and heavy metal concentrations were determined using UNICAM-929 spectrophotometry device.

Results: In spite of no significant differences in terms of average zinc (Zn) concentration, height, or weight between cases and controls, significant differences were noted for manganese (Mn), lead (Pb), cadmium (Cd), magnesium (Mg), iron (Fe), copper (Cu) and cobalt (Co) ($p < 0.05$).

Conclusion: This study suggests that heavy metals may play an etiological role in the occurrence of chronic TE. However, contrary to previous studies, Zn did not appear to play an important causative role, while these subjects had increased serum Fe levels.

COMMENT

Telogen effluvium (TE) is the most frequent cause of hair loss and is associated with diffuse and nonscarring hair loss. Essential heavy metals are associated with beneficial effects in humans as well as in other living organisms. However, they may lead to toxic effects when the exposure exceeds the higher tolerable limits. The potential routes of entry of heavy metals into the body include either natural environmental exposure or other means such as mining, soil erosion, industrial waste, air pollution or pesticides. Although occupational exposure is possible in some individuals, diet represents the major source of exposure. In this study, they examined the levels of trace elements including iron (Fe), zinc (Zn), manganese (Mn), copper (Cu) and magnesium (Mg) as well as the levels of heavy metals such as cobalt (Co), cadmium (Cd) and lead (Pb) in patients with chronic TE and compared them with that of control subjects. In addition to above, clinicians should also look into the possibility of patient taking homeopathy medicines with high potencies over a long period of time, as homeopathy medicines contain metals as active ingredients.

Contrary to previously held belief, Zn did not appear to be an important etiological factor, and serum Fe levels were elevated in the chronic TE group. Significant increase in Fe levels as compared to controls seems to imply that Fe supplementation may actually be counterproductive rather than providing benefit. Cigarette smoking represents the most important nonoccupational cause of Cd exposure. Smokers have significantly elevated Cd levels in blood, urine, hair and other tissues as compared to nonsmokers leading to hair loss. In the current study, serum Mg levels were significantly low in TE patients, suggesting that Mg supplementation may be used against hair loss, particularly in healthy individuals. Pb may play an etiologic role in the development of chronic TE, even without toxic exposure levels. In this study, patients had higher serum Cu levels than controls; this may indicate a need to reassess the role of Cu supplementation used for hair loss treatment. Patients with TE had a significant elevation in their Mn and Co levels.

Small sample size is the major limitation in this study. Further studies are required to better delineate the association between hair loss and trace elements as well as heavy metals.

> **Key Messages**
> - Heavy metals may play a causative role in the occurrence of chronic TE
> - Contrary to previously held belief, Zn did not appear to be an important etiological factor of chronic TE
> - To keep an eye on possible etiology of TE from usage of home remedies and alternative medicines like ayurveda homeopathy siddha and unani.

ARTICLE 105

Reduced Ferritin, Folate and Vitamin B12 Levels in Female Patients Diagnosed with Telogen Effluvium

Ertug EY, Yilmaz RA. Reduced ferritin, folate, and vitamin B12 levels in female patients diagnosed with telogen effluvium. *Int J Med Biochem. 2018;1(3):111-4.*

Abstract

Objectives: Telogen effluvium (TE) is the most common cause of diffuse hair shedding. It is a noninflammatory process characterized by the widespread loss of hair follicles in the telogen phase. Identification of its etiology requires laboratory tests involving endocrine, nutritional, and autoimmune disorders, and detailed anamnesis. The aim of this study was to examine serum ferritin, folate and vitamin B12 levels in female patients with TE, and to investigate their possible role in the disease pathogenesis.

Methods: The study included 651 female patients: 455 in the TE group and 196 in the control group. Serum ferritin, folate and vitamin B12 levels were measured in both the groups.

Results: Patients with TE had significantly lower serum ferritin concentrations compared to those in the control group (17.35 ± 18.54 ng/mL vs. 39.27 ± 29.44 ng/mL) (p = 0.001). The folate levels were significantly lower in the TE group compared to those in the control group (7.94 ± 8.98 ng/mL vs. 11.31 ± 4.7 ng/mL) (p = 0.001). Vitamin B12 concentrations were also significantly lower in the TE group (232.13 ± 123.35 pg/mL) (p = 0.001).

Conclusion: It was concluded that reduced levels of ferritin, vitamin B12 and folate might play a role in development of TE.

COMMENT

This is a case-control study which included 455 female patients aged between 18 and 45 years and diagnosed with Telogen effluvium (TE) by detailed clinical examination. The control group consisted of 198 female patients who presented to the outpatient clinic for nevus treatment and did not complain of hair loss.

Serum iron, hemoglobin (Hb), ferritin, folate and vitamin B12 concentrations in TE and control groups were compared against the reference intervals. For female patients, the reference intervals were 60-180 µg/dL for iron, 10.8-15.1 g/dL for Hb, 11-306 ng/mL for ferritin, 5.2-20 ng/mL for folate and 180-914 pg/mL for vitamin B12. Ferritin, folate and vitamin B12 levels were measured with sandwich immunoenzymatic method.

In this study, serum ferritin, iron, folate and vitamin B12 levels were significantly lower in the TE patients. There was weak correlation between age and folate and vitamin B12 levels. There was weak correlation between ferritin levels and vitamin B12; folate and vitamin B12 levels. Reduced ferritin and iron deficiency is an important risk factor for the TE development.

The differences between the studies regarding iron, ferritin and Hb levels may have multifactorial reasons. The variations in the results may depend on the behavioral habits in the society such as insufficient iron intake and reduced iron absorption because of excess consumption of tea and coffee. Although ferritin is the best indicator of iron deficiency, in unreliable conditions such as chronic inflammation, infection, neoplasia or renal failure, confirmatory tests may be needed.

The role of folate and vitamin B12 in hair growth is unknown. In this study, their levels were significantly low in TE patients.

Key Messages

- The two most important investigations ordered for TE patients are serum ferritin and thyroid profile
- In case of TE with low ferritin levels, it is worthwhile administering iron preparations preferably by intravenous infusion, as absorption of iron through oral administration could be poor in severely depleted patients
- Low levels of ferritin, vitamin B12 and folate might play a role in the TE development. Hence patients with TE should be evaluated for these parameters, too in case of non-response to iron supplementation alone.

ARTICLE 106

Color-transition Sign: A Useful Trichoscopic Finding for Differentiating Alopecia Areata Incognita from Telogen Effluvium

Kinoshita-Ise M, Fukuyama M, Ohyama M. Color-transition sign: A useful trichoscopic finding for differentiating alopecia areata incognita from telogen effluvium.
J Dermatol. 2018;45(8):e224-5.

Abstract

Alopecia areata incognita (AAI), also known as diffuse alopecia areata, is a variant of alopecia areata (AA) described predominantly in young women. It is characterized by abrupt and intense hair loss without typical alopecic patches. This disease presentation closely resembles that of telogen effluvium (TE). Color-transition sign, a useful trichoscopic finding, helps in differentiating AAI from TE.

COMMENT

Alopecia areata incognito (AAI) is a variant of alopecia areata (AA) with diffuse hair loss misdiagnosed as telogen effluvium (TE). Histopathologic findings of AAI are similar to AA. Scalp biopsy is invasive and sometimes impractical, especially for pediatric cases. Trichoscopic detection of tapering hair, broken hair, black dots and yellow dots characteristic of AA can hardly be detectable in AAI. This article reports a case of AAI with distinct dermoscopic finding to differentiate AAI from TE. In AAI, trichoscopy showed brighter brownish color at their proximal portion due to cornified proximal roots demonstrating color graduation from black to clear between the distal end and the proximal root. This trichoscopic finding is named as "color-transition sign", which suggests a relatively long-standing assault on bulbs of hair follicles.

In AA, melanocyte-associated antigens are suggested to be targets of autoreactive cytotoxic T lymphocytes. Inflammation in AAI is speculated to be milder than typical AA. This inflammation can be insufficient to trigger rapid anagen–telogen conversion allowing anagen hair to grow but enough to impair the hair shaft pigmentation process leading to this trichoscopic finding.

Key Message

- The color-transition sign, brownish discoloration at their proximal portion detected by trichoscopy seen in AAI, can be a distinct finding in differentiating AAI from TE. Further accumulation of such cases is required as it differentiates AAI from TE for better management of this unusual subset of AA.

ARTICLE 107

Trichoscopy in Pediatric Age Group

Malakar S, Mehta PR, Mukherjee SS. Trichoscopy in pediatric age group.
Indian J Paediatr Dermatol. 2018;19:93-101.

Abstract

Trichoscope is a noninvasive tool helpful in the diagnosis of trichological disorders; improves the diagnostic and clinical acumen of the clinicians. It serves as a prognostic and monitoring tool in therapeutic management with pattern analysis ranging from hair shaft patterns to follicular, perifollicular and interfollicular patterns. The article describes trichoscopic features of noncicatricial alopecias, cicatricial alopecias and genetic hair shaft defects compiled with a Fotofinder, DermLite Foto II Pro and DermLite DL 3N dermoscopes.

COMMENT

The trichoscopic patterns are analyzed in a systematic way, initially observing changes in hair shaft, followed by follicular, perifollicular and interfollicular pattern. Understanding normal changes, like vellus hair appears hypopigmented and nonmedullated and terminal hair is uniform in color and thickness along its entire length, forms the basics of trichoscopy. Hair shaft changes described are tapering hair, exclamation hair, circle/pigtail hair, Pohl-Pinkus constriction, regrowing hair, comma hair, corkscrew hair, Z hair, broken hair, flame hair, block hair, I hair and coiled hair. Follicular patterns include black dots, yellow dots, white dots, red dots, blue-gray dots, keratotic plugs while perifollicular findings are scales, hair casts and peripilar sign. Interfollicular patterns include honeycomb pigment network, interfollicular scales and red loops, and white patches.

The article also describes trichoscopic points that favor scarring alopecia over a nonscarring alopecia. Triad of absence of hair follicle openings, whitish structureless areas and presence of milky red areas indicating recent onset fibrosis points toward scarring alopecia.

Findings in nonscarring alopecia: In alopecia areata, yellow dots, black dots, tapered hair, broken hair, vellus hair and Pohl-Pinkus constriction are often seen; exclamation mark hair, black dots and broken hair are markers for disease activity. Short regrowing hair and pigtail hair indicate hair regrowth. In trichotillomania, flame hair, tulip hair, I hair, block hair, V sign, mace hair and hair powder are seen; "burnt matchstick sign" has also been described. Tinea capitis shows comma and corkscrew hair, Morse-code hair, broken hair, black dots, I hair, block hair and hair casts. Telogen effluvium shows short regrowing hair, empty follicles, while anagen effluvium shows yellow dots, black dots, tapering hair, Pohl-Pinkus constriction, circle hair, tulip hair-like structure or tulipoid hair and peripilar sign. Patterned hair loss shows anisotrichosis >20%, yellow dots, vellus hair, peripilar sign and decreased number of hair emerging per follicular unit. In congenital triangular alopecia, cluster of short vellus hair with diversity in length is seen.

Cicatricial alopecia: In discoid lupus erythematosus, follicular keratotic openings, disruption of the honeycomb pattern resulting in loss of pigment, perifollicular and interfollicular blue-gray dots, loss of follicular openings, thick arborizing vessels and red dots are seen. Lichen planopilaris shows perifollicular scaling, peripilar casts, tufting of 2-3 hair, perifollicular blue-gray dots in a target pattern, milky red areas, fibrotic white patches, absence of follicular openings, and absence of vellus hair. Hair tufts with yellow scales, collar formation, and epidermal hyperplasia in the perifollicular region seen as a star burst pattern are seen in dissecting cellulitis of scalp.

In scalp infestation, common in pediatric age, trichoscopy can be helpful. Lice, viable nits and pseudonits can be well visualized. Trichoscopy can be useful in genetic hair shaft defects like trichorrhexis nodosa (gray–white areas and the classical paintbrush bristle appearance), trichorrhexis invaginata (tiny nodules), monilithrix (multiple beaded hair with nodes and internodes placed equidistant), pili torti (multiple twists along the hair shaft), pili annulati (transverse bands cloudy white in color), loose anagen hair syndrome (decreased number of terminal hair, empty follicles and primarily single follicle hair units) and congenital atrichia with papules ("cluster of stars" appearance).

Trichoscopy also guides for biopsy; it can be utilized to choose an appropriate area for a biopsy.

> **Key Messages**
> - Basic trichoscopic and characteristic trichoscopic features of common trichological conditions can help in diagnosis, treatment, management and also follow-up
> - Considering the intricacies of investigations like biopsy, trichoscope for evaluation among pediatric age group is a magnificent tool and avoids biopsy in the majority of pediatric hair disorders. Trichoscopy is a tool to reckon with, not only in adults but also more importantly in children.

ARTICLE 108

Dermoscopic Findings in Psoriasis and Seborrheic Dermatitis on the Scalp and Correlation with Disease Severity

Ficicioglu S, Piskin S. Dermoscopic findings in psoriasis and seborrheic dermatitis on the scalp and correlation with disease severity.
Med-Science. 2018;7(1):118-21.

Abstract

Dermoscopy has frequently been used for hair and scalp disorders. Dermoscopic examinations of psoriasis and seborrheic dermatitis lesions yielded different morphologies. This study aimed to investigate the usefulness of dermoscopy in the clinical differentiation of psoriasis and seborrheic dermatitis on the scalp and additionally to evaluate its capacity in determining disease severity. The study included 46 psoriasis and 50 seborrheic dermatitis patients who were clinically diagnosed and had scalp lesions. Dermoscopic images taken from lesional scalp were then reviewed for microvascular patterns. In addition, we assessed the severity of scalp disease and looked for a correlation with these patterns. The frequency of twisted loops, glomerular vessels, red dots/globules and polymorphous beaded lines/circles were statistically higher in the psoriasis group, whereas the frequencies of simple loops and arborizing vessels were statistically higher in the seborrheic dermatitis group (p <0.001). There was no significant difference in the frequency of featureless areas between two groups (p = 0.579). There was no correlation with disease severity and dermoscopic findings. In conclusion, dermoscopy is a valuable and easy-to-use tool for differentiating psoriasis and seborrheic dermatitis on the scalp even if it does not have enough strength to determine disease severity. In addition, there is some diversity and ambiguity concerning terminology, which can be resolved with future studies and the establishment of conventional terms.

COMMENT

Psoriasis and seborrheic dermatitis are inflammatory skin diseases with erythematous squamous lesions, and sometimes it might be extremely difficult to differentiate between these two, even with histopathological evaluation. Dermoscopy is a noninvasive, practical tool helpful in diagnosis of dermatological conditions. This study was based on the diagnosis of psoriasis and seborrheic dermatitis on the scalp by using dermoscope, and also correlating it with disease severity.

In this study, the patients with psoriasis and seborrheic dermatitis were evaluated for the appearance of vascular structures and featureless areas. Psoriasis Scalp Severity Index (PSSI) and Seborrheic Dermatitis Scalp Severity Index (SDSSI) were utilized to assess the disease severity.

There were higher frequencies of simple loops and arborizing vessels in seborrheic dermatitis compared to psoriasis. The frequencies of twisted loops, glomerular vessels, red dots/globules and polymorphous beaded lines/circles were higher in the psoriasis than in the seborrheic dermatitis group. No difference between groups for featureless areas. These findings seen in this article were compatible with the literature. There was no relationship between the scalp disease severity indexes (PSSI, SDSSI) and the study findings.

The small sample size and inclusion of only scalp limits this study.

Dermoscope is an easy-to-use tool which can be utilized in differentiation of scaly scalp lesions, especially where the two important disease to be ruled out are psoriasis and seborrheic dermatitis. The presence of particular visual structures through dermoscope decreases the need for biopsy and histopathological evaluation.

Key Messages

- Before using the dermoscope, the affected part has to be cleaned and scales to be dislodged
- Dermoscopy can be useful in differentiating psoriasis and seborrheic dermatitis, as it allows to apprehend morphological structures that are otherwise invisible to the naked eye
- The need for biopsy will decrease, and it will be possible to obtain objective data during therapy
- Dermoscope cannot be utilized to determine disease severity, but can be used to assess response to treatment.

ARTICLE 109

Utility of Trichoscopy in Tinea Capitis

Daroach M, Hanumanthu V, Kumaran MS. Utility of trichoscopy in tinea capitis.
Postgrad Med J. 2019;95(1121):173.

Abstract

Dermoscope, also called as skin surface microscope or epiluminescence microscope, is a simple noninvasive tool used in the diagnosis of skin lesions. Here we present a case report of a 7-year-old, presenting with history of grayish patchy hair loss. The occurrence of typical trichoscopic features aided in the diagnosis of tinea capitis obviating the need of other investigations. The very use of trichoscope as a simple tool in diagnosis has been highlighted in this article.

COMMENT

Dermoscope, also called as skin surface microscope or epiluminescence microscope, is a simple noninvasive tool used in the diagnosis of skin condition. This article highlights the importance of use of dermoscope in common clinical conditions like tinea capitis for quicker and accurate diagnosis of the condition.

The author has presented a case report of a 7-year-old, presenting with history of grayish patchy hair loss associated with itching seen at Dermatology Department, PGIMER, Chandigarh. The occurrence of comma-shaped hair, corkscrew hair and black dots confirmed the diagnosis of tinea capitis. This helped in obviating the need for histopathological examination or even 10% KOH wet mount in its diagnosis.

Trichoscope helps to visualize the epidermis, dermo-epidermal junction and dermis. It aids dermatologists to clinically diagnose conditions without the need of lengthy and/or invasive procedures. It is also helpful in epidemiological surveys and health camps where laboratory facilities would not be easily available. The very use of trichoscope as a simple tool in diagnosis has been highlighted in this article.

Key Messages

- Trichoscope is a simple, noninvasive, innovative tool which helps in diagnosis of common scalp disorder with more accuracy, without the need for high-end machines or lengthy/invasive procedures
- Trichoscope is a boon in endemic outreach areas and health camps where laboratory facilities are not easily available. It can also be used in busy clinics where lengthy diagnostic procedures are not possible.

ARTICLE 110

Dermoscopy for Discriminating between Trichophyton and Microsporum Infections in Tinea Capitis

Lekkas D, Ioannides D, Apalla Z, et al. Dermoscopy for discriminating between Trichophyton and Microsporum infections in tinea capitis.
J Eur Acad Dermatol Venereol. 2018;32(6):e234-5.

Abstract

Dermoscopy aids the clinical recognition of tinea capitis (TC) and specific dermoscopic criteria have been associated with its diagnosis (black dots, comma hair, corkscrew hair etc.). This article provides data on correlation between dermoscopic structures and the genera of the causative fungi.

COMMENT

A 3-year-old and a 7-year-old boy presented with the scalp lesions suggestive of tinea capitis (TC) clinically. Dermoscopic examination was performed and dermoscopic images were captured.

Dermoscopy of the first patient revealed black dots, comma hair and corkscrew hair, and minimal perifollicular scales. In second patient, there was presence of prominent scale and Morse code-like hair along with broken hair. The KOH examination and fungal culture confirmed diagnosis of TC with causative agents as *Trichophyton tonsurans* and *Microsporum canis*. Morse code-like hair represent multiple horizontal white bands with normal looking hair keratin between them. These white bands represent localized areas of fungal infection with large density of hyphae and arthroconidia. Black dots correlate with cadaverised hair and comma hair correlate with broken hair which result from cracking and bending of hair shaft due to hyphae. Corkscrew hair is considered as variation of the comma hair and represent broken coiled hair and they are result of a specific type of fungi. This paper concludes that Morse code-like hair could be due to ectothrix type of parasitation and suggests *Microsporum* infection, as trichophyta rarely causes ectothrix parasitation.

Key Messages

- *Different dermoscopic features can aid in diagnosing the genera of the causative fungi*
- *Morse-code hair may be indicative of ectothrix infection suggestive of Microsporum.*

ARTICLE 111

A Prospective Study of Tinea Capitis in Children: Making the Diagnosis Easier with a Dermoscope

Aqil A, BayBay H, Moustaide K, et al. A prospective study of tinea capitis in children: Making the diagnosis easier with a dermoscope.
J Med Case Rep. 2018;12(1):383.

Abstract

A prospective descriptive analytical study of 34 children with tinea capitis (TC) was conducted with trichoscopic examination of all patients; with mycological culture done in only six children. Trichoscopy showed hair shaft abnormalities in all cases and hence authors have proposed a classification of trichoscopic signs of TC. The classification enables rapid diagnosis and prediction of the type of fungus before mycological culture, to facilitate early institution of treatment.

COMMENT

Trichoscopy is a simple, fast, economical, and bedside tool available for diagnosing and monitoring tinea capitis (TC) in children. Dermoscopic signs specific to TC have prompted the authors to classify TC depending on the clinical patterns as microsporic TC, trichophytic TC or inflammatory TC and also find a correlation between the dermoscopic signs and the clinical subtype. The study recruited 34 children with alopecic plaques suggestive of TC. The average mean age was found to be 8.42 years (3–14 years) comprising of 67.6% boys and 32.4% girls, with a sex ratio of 2.09. Microsporic TC was seen in 47.51%, trichophytic TC in 29.4% and inflammatory TC in 23.5%. Dermoscope signs observed were mainly broken hair in 91.2%, 82.4% showed follicular keratosis, 85.3% had scales, black dots in 73.5%, while bent hair was found in 70.6%, erythema in 64.7%, comma hair and crusts were seen in 55.9% and 50%, respectively. Corkscrew hair were seen in 35.3%, forked hair in 32.4% while bar code-like hair was noted in 26.5%. Follicular pustules were seen in 23.5% and zigzag hair in 17.6%, also translucent hair was seen in 11.8% and V-shaped hair in 11.8%. Corkscrew hair was significantly present in female children ($p < 0.05$, $r = 0.016$) in univariate analysis with comma hair and corkscrew hair in microsporic TC ($p < 0.001$, $r = 0.685$ and $p < 0.05$, $r = 0.536$, respectively), inflammatory TC mainly showed V-shaped hair ($p < 0.05$, $r = 0.017$); and crusts and follicular pustules ($p < 0.05$, $r = 0.061$ and $p < 0.001$, $r = 0.000$, respectively), scales and follicular keratosis in noninflammatory TC ($p < 0.001$, $r = 0.000$ and $p < 0.05$, $r = 0.038$, respectively), and finally, in trichophytic and inflammatory TC erythema was seen ($p < 0.001$, $r = 0.889$).

Thus, in conclusion, comma hair and corkscrew hair were dominant dermoscopic features in microsporic TC; V-shaped hair in inflammatory tinea capitis; on the contrary, noninflammatory TC showed scales and follicular keratosis and inflammatory TC had crusts and follicular pustules. In trichophytic and inflammatory TC, erythema was characteristic. The specificity of these corkscrew hair and comma hair signs in TC was well established in the study since they disappeared during the course of treatment. Authors also state that corkscrew hair could be a variant of comma hair in black patients or a specificity of TC due to *Trichophyton soudanense*; the authors believe that since the study group was intermediate skin phototype; higher prevalence of these two signs was appreciated.

However, larger prospective studies with mycological culture are needed to confirm this classification as mycological confirmation (direct examination and culture) was not available for all patients in the study.

Key Message

- Trichoscopy helps not only in diagnosis but also monitoring of tinea capitis.

ARTICLE 112

Tinea Capitis in Children: A Report of Four Cases with Trichoscopic Features

Elghblawi E. Tinea capitis in children: A report of four cases trichoscopic with trichoscopic features. *Indian J Paediatr Dermatol. 2018;19:51-6.*

Abstract

Tinea capitis (TC) is the superficial dermatophyte infection commonly seen in pediatric population with ethnic variation of causative species. Fungal culture is the gold standard investigation but trichoscopy aids a speedy diagnosis by its characteristic findings. Scalp dermoscopy or "trichoscopy" represents a valuable, noninvasive technique for the evaluation of patients with hair loss due to TC. The article presents four reported cases of TC from different locations, background, and geography, and the role of dermoscopy in diagnosis.

COMMENT

Tinea capitis (TC) is the superficial dermatophyte infection commonly seen in pediatric population with ethnic variation of causative species. Fungal culture is the gold standard investigation but trichoscopy aids a speedy diagnosis by its characteristic findings. Scalp dermoscopy or "trichoscopy" represents a valuable, noninvasive technique for the evaluation of patients with hair loss due to TC. The article presents four reported cases of TC from different locations, background, and geography and the role of dermoscopy in diagnosis.

Case 1: A 14-year-old child from Libya had slightly pruritic scalp lesions from past 2 months and was treated with corticosteroids; frequent contact with animals and cats with unidentified skin disease was present. An erythematous scaly, partially alopecic, plaque on the right parietal region characterized by superficial crusts was seen. Woods lamp showed green fluorescent hair. No dermoscopy was done. Oral griseofulvin at a dosage of 10 mg/kg/day for 8–12 weeks was started and the complete clinical resolution was seen at 4 months follow-up with no evidence of residual scarring alopecia.

Case 2: A 5-year-old Libyan male child had a crusted plaque on his scalp of 6 weeks with no prior topical or systemic treatment. A crusted, nonerythematous, rounded lesion on the parietal area of the head showed blue fluorescence on Woods lamp. Trichoscopy showed comma hair, corkscrew hair (CH), zigzag hair and a bar code hair. (Contact-type DermLite PRO II and connected with iPhone 4S, with alcohol as the interface medium used) oral terbinafine (125 mg/day) for 6 weeks was prescribed.

Case 3: An 8-year-old male child from Sudan, skin phototype 5, was presented with a 2-month history of two patches of crusted, noninflammatory lesions on his occipital scalp. Fine, whitish scale on the scalp with alopecia patches had hair fragility on the hair pull test and showed green fluorescence under the Woods lamp. Dermoscopy revealed numerous broken-down hair as well as hair with a distinguishing comma-like shape [consistent and homogenous thickness and color and marked distal angulation (3Gen DermLite with Olympus bridge camera used)] Topical and oral terbinafine was given.

Case 4: A 6-year-old Turkish girl had a single pruritic plaque of alopecia on the right side of her scalp for 3 weeks and contact with a cat. The hair pull test was positive. KOH mount was positive. On dermoscopic examination, there were multiple hair with a characteristic comma shape (DL4 dermoscope with a Nikon camera used). The condition resolved with 8 weeks treatment of oral ketoconazole at ¼ TSF twice per day.

Dermoscopy in TC shows mainly two typical features, comma and CH. The main observed trichoscopic findings were comma hair and zigzag hair in three patients. Broken or black dots and dystrophic hair were not seen; Morse code hair was noted in Case 2. Hair slightly curved and fractured hair shaft is described as a dermatoscopic marker for TC in white children with *Microsporum canis* infection and CH as additional feature in Trichophyton or Microsporum infection. Authors propose that CH is not a peculiar manifestation in black patients but rather a possible manifestation related to curly hair. Case series also highlights the anthropophilic nature of TC. No mycological study was done in the cases which is a major drawback. The standard treatment is griseofulvin and traditional drug of choice; however, itraconazole (3 mg/kg/day to 5 mg/kg/day for 4-6 weeks) and terbinafine (62.5-250 mg/day for 4 weeks) have replaced it successfully.

Key Messages

- *Dermoscopy forms a rapid and magnified in vivo visualization of the hair and scalp skin; reduces the need for scalp biopsy and useful for monitoring, treatment and follow-up*
- *Comma hair were observed as a distinctive trichoscopic feature of proposed M. canis-induced TC*
- *Dermoscopy reduces the need for KOH mount and fungal culture, particularly useful in community dermatology camps and a busy OPD.*

Section 6 Surgical Trichology

ARTICLE 113

Study of Efficacy and Safety of Noncultured, Extracted Follicular Outer Root Sheath Cell Suspension Transplantation in the Management of Stable Vitiligo

Kumar P, Bhari N, Tembhre MK, et al. Study of efficacy and safety of noncultured, extracted follicular outer root sheath cell suspension transplantation in the management of stable vitiligo.
Int J Dermatol. 2018;57(2):245-9.

Abstract

A recent introduction in the treatment of stable vitiligo is the use of noncultured, extracted follicular outer root sheath cell suspension (NC-EHF-ORS-CS) technique. This study was done with an objective to find the clinical efficacy of this technique and to determine the cell composition and viability of the suspension. It included 25 stable vitiligo patients. From each patient, 50 follicles were extracted from the occipital area and incubated with trypsin–ethylene diamine tetraacetic acid to separate outer root sheath cells. The cell suspension thus obtained was applied to dermabraded recipient site. The viability of cell suspension was checked using trypan blue staining and markers of keratinocyte stem cells (CD200) and melanocytes (S100) were evaluated with flow cytometry and immunocytochemistry. The results showed that, at the end of 6 months, mean repigmentation was $52 \pm 25.1\%$ and 8/32 (32%) patients showed >75% repigmentation. The mean percentage cell viability of suspension was $80 \pm 17.2\%$ with mean concentration of CD200+ and S100+ cells being $7.91 \pm 8.68\%$ and $9.93 \pm 1.22\%$ (n = 3), respectively. Four out of 25 (16%) patients showed recipient site infection and a color mismatch was observed in 11 out of 25 (44%) patients. The study concluded with NC-EHF-ORS-CS as a useful minimally invasive therapy for treating vitiligo.

COMMENT

Various surgical techniques have been devised over the years for treatment of resistant and stable vitiligo cases with variable response. Hence there is a continuous search for a better technique for the surgical management of vitiligo. The hair follicle stem cells is new arena.

The outer root sheath of the hair follicle contains stem cells of melanocytes and keratinocyte lineages capable of differentiation. Hair follicle melanocytes are more active, more numerous, larger and immunologically privileged. The melanocyte-keratinocyte ratio in hair follicle is 1:1-1:6 as compared to

1:36 in epidermis and hair follicle stem cells show higher propensity to proliferate toward melanocyte lineage. These make hair follicle a very attractive source of melanocytes for transplantation in vitiligo.

There were 25 patients in this study. Fifty follicles were extracted from occipital scalp of each patient. These follicles were incubated with trypsin-ethylene diaminetetraacetic acid to separate outer root sheath cells. The cell suspension obtained was subjected to filtration and centrifugation to get a cell pellet. The pellet was resuspended and applied to the recipient area after dermabrasion. The cell viability of the suspension was assessed using trypan blue staining. The evaluation of the markers of keratinocyte stem cells (CD200) and melanocytes (S100) was done using flow cytometry and immunocytochemistry, respectively.

At the end of 6 months, the mean (SD) repigmentation was $52 \pm 25.1\%$ and 8/25 (32%) patients had shown >75% repigmentation. The cell viability of the suspension was having mean percentage of $80 \pm 17.2\%$. The mean concentration of CD200+ and S100+ cells being $7.91 \pm 8.68\%$ and $9.93 \pm 1.22\%$ (n = 3), respectively.

The repigmentation was further analyzed according to the type of vitiligo and differences in the improvement in the different forms of vitiligo at the 1st, 3rd and 6th month of follow-up were not statistically significant. The results were good on head and neck compared to acral lesions. This technique has fewer donor site complications in comparison to the conventional epidermal cell suspension technique.

In a similar open-label, prospective, comparative study by Donaparthi et al. 11 patients having 60 stable vitiligo sites were treated with epidermal melanocyte transfer (EMT) and extracted hair follicular outer root sheath cell transfer (HFMT). In the results, at the end of 6 months, >90% repigmentation was seen in 83.33% patches of EMT group and 43.33% in HFMT group. Ninety percent of patches in the epidermal group and 43.34% of patches in the hair follicular group have shown >75% repigmentation respectively.

In an another similar comparative study by Singh et al. involving 30 patients with 47 stable vitiligo lesions, the extent of repigmentation was excellent (90–100%) in 83% of lesions in the noncultured epidermal cell suspension group and 65% of lesions in the NC-EHF-ORS-CS group.

The repigmentation depends upon the number of hair follicle stem cells and melanocytes transplanted to recipient sites. So to increase the yield, type I collagenase enzyme can be added in the solution which results in lysis of perifollicular dermal sheath resulting in better penetration of trypsin into outer root sheath of hair follicle. Thus NC-EHF-ORS-CS transplantation is a good technique with a good yield of melanocytes for the surgical management of stable vitiligo. But the superiority of this technique in achieving repigmentation compared to NCECS is yet to be established by further studies.

Key Messages

- The HFSC are active and immune privileged cells in bulge region that are responsible for perifollicular repigmentation
- The NC-EHF-ORS-CS transplantation is a good minimally invasive technique and is having a good yield of melanocytes for management of stable vitiligo with surgery
- The donor site complications are less with this technique as compared to conventional epidermal cell suspension technique.

ARTICLE 114

Controversies in Hair Transplantation

Kumaresan M, Mysore V. Controversies in Hair Transplantation.
J Cutan Aesthet Surg. 2018;11(4):173-81.

Abstract
A relatively newer field being hair transplantation (HT), several aspects raise controversies and issues. The issues refer to both evidence and ethics and how community and the practitioners need to deal with them. This article highlights few of such diverse issues as safe donor area, platelet-rich plasma (PRP), follicular unit extraction versus follicular unit transplantation and minimum qualification required for performing HT.

COMMENT

Platelet-rich plasma (PRP) is used extensively in hair transplantation (HT). PRP, Platelet rich fibrin matrix (PRFM), Plasma rich in growth factors (PRGF) and Platelet lysate (PL) have been claimed to have therapeutic effectiveness for androgenetic alopecia (AGA). Its use in hair transplantation to enhance the results is debatable.

Platelet-rich plasma has been used in the following steps in HT:
- As a holding solution for the grafts
- Injecting PRP in the recipient area before making the incisions
- Injecting into the recipient area immediately after making the slits
- Topical application over the grafted site
- At end of surgery immediately after implantation of grafts, injected into the recipient area
- After surgery, injection into the recipient area in several sessions (over months) to increase the growth of grafted hairs.

To augment surgical procedures, PRP appears to be a promising treatment. The literature reported so far, though less, have documented the decrease in catagen hair loss postoperatively following HT. PRP/PRFM/PL/PRGF can enhance results by improving the skin milieu of grafted area by cell growth and differentiation, anti-apoptotic activity and neovascularization, making grafted area more receptive and fertile for newly transplanted hair.

However, large studies are needed for the desired platelet count, quantity, duration, interval between the sessions and the mode of application.

Safe donor area (SDA)—Occipital scalp hair, being androgen resistant, has taken over as the donor area. In production of satisfactory outcome in HT, efficient utilization of donor zone remains the most important factor. SDA has not been clear cut defined and there are differences in races. New concepts such as diffuse AGA, reverse pattern hair loss and possibility of miniaturization in occipital scalp have also come in light. Many SDAs have been proposed over the time like Ungers

SDA, Cole's SDA, Bernstein and Rassman SDA and Park's whorl theory. However, it is worth stating that there cannot be one valid, totally safe donor zone for all patients. Assessment of future progression of AGA, a family history, and clinical examination would be required to confirm the SDA boundaries. The lower and upper limits of donor area should not be breached as harvesting nonsafe hair leads to future loss from the grafted area which is unethical and would bring the technique into disrepute.

Follicular unit transplantation (FUT) versus follicular unit extraction (FUE)—FUE and strip harvesting are both acceptable techniques for donor grafts harvesting. Both techniques have disadvantages as well as advantage. Combining FUE and FUT improves the yield and graft outcome. When multiple sessions of HT are required, FUT scores more, and also when to have maximum number of the grafts from SDA. For the patients who insist for not having a linear scar, FUE is well suited. FUE is an excellent choice for small procedure seeking young patients. For harvesting leg, trunk and arm hair, FUE is an excellent option and it has an advantage to camouflage strip scars. However, unqualified people have started doing this procedure independently due to simplicity of this technique, without surgeon's supervision. Surgeons should know all surgical types and should use the technique best suited for each patient.

Who should perform hair transplant surgery? According to the International Society of Hair Restoration Surgery (ISHRS), any procedure that has tissue removal from the body or scalp, by any means, must be done by a licensed physician in the field of medicine. Physicians who perform hair restoration surgery (HRS) must possess the training, education and current competency in the field of HRS. The nonlicensed personnel should not perform surgery. The internationally accepted guidelines, also endorsed by the Association of Hair Restoration Surgeons (AHRS)-India, in regards to role of a hair transplant surgeon, states that the following steps of HRS should be performed by a hair transplant surgeon who is qualified:

- Preoperative consultation and diagnostic evaluation
- Surgery execution and planning including:
  - Harvesting donor hair
  - Designing hairline
  - Creation of recipient site
  - Management of possible adverse reaction and other patient medical issues
  - Postoperative care.

The AHRS-India in October, 2015 has resolved that the only specialties eligible to become members of AHRS-India would be:

- The master of plastic surgery
- Doctor of medicine or postgraduate in dermatology
- Master of surgery (MS) or postgraduate in ear nose throat surgery
- MS general surgery.

The technicians assisting in hair restoration surgeries should not perform any aspect of surgery independently. They are allowed to perform only those steps, which do not involve incision of the body under supervision of a physician. Hence, they should not perform incision (scoring), suturing and slit making. They can be involved in extraction of the grafts after incision, premade slit implantation, grafts arrangement and postoperative dressings.

> **Key Messages**
> - Hair transplantation being a relatively newer field, several aspects raise issues and controversies
> - Debatable issues such as FUT versus FUE, SDA and PRP are chosen based on knowledge and discretion of the operating surgeon
> - The physician must be fulfilling the criteria for qualifying to perform a HRS in order to be ethical in practice and to avoid legal complications.

ARTICLE 115

Adipose Tissue Transplant in Recurrent Folliculitis Decalvans

Tedesco M. Adipose tissue transplant in recurrent folliculitis decalvans.
Int J Immunopathol Pharmacol. 2018;32:1-4.

Abstract

Folliculitis decalvans (FD) is a rare primary neutrophilic scarring alopecia. This article reports the use of autologous fat transplantation (AFT) as a source of stem cell therapy for hair regrowth in FD. After treatment with AFT, the patient had no new pustules and no longer had pain or burning sensation in the affected area with clinical improvement.

COMMENT

Folliculitis decalvans (FD), primary neutrophilic scarring alopecia occurs in young and middle-aged adults, with a higher prevalence in the male gender. *Staphylococcus aureus* and genetic predisposition seem to play an important role in this pathogenesis with the overall incidence of 11% mainly involving vertex and occipital area. FD is associated with itching, pain, and/or burning sensations. Tufted hair folliculitis is characteristic due to the damage of the follicle infundibular epithelium with the formation of the common infundibulum.

The current treatment includes systemic antibiotics, oral isotretinoin, topical and intralesional steroids, biologics, photodynamic therapy, and lasers (Nd-Yag). The surgical option should be carefully chosen in such cases. In this case report, autologous fat transplantation (AFT) is used as a source of stem cell for hair regrowth assisted by the inflammatory action of fat. In literature, fat grafting is used to accelerate hair regrowth, but no data as curative in FD.

In the study, a 41-year-old Caucasian female patient with prolong history of FD underwent two sessions of AFT 5 months apart using 20 mL of fat emulsion injected 0.2 cc/cm². (Though there is no information about depth of injections and also gauge of needle or cannula used) After treatment, there were no new folliculitis and had no pain or burning sensation in the area affected. Hair regrowth could already be seen in the peripheral region of the affected area. The limitation being that the follow-up duration is not mentioned and also whether one treatment session is enough to have sustainable results. This report insights larger studies with longer follow-up to prove the efficacy of adipose tissue transplant as curative.

Key Messages
- Folliculitis decalvans is a chronic scarring alopecia often resistant to conventional and combined treatments
- Adipose tissue transplant is used to accelerate hair regrowth in the literature
- Adipose tissue is used as a stem cell for its anti-inflammatory and regenerative effect, though there are no studies regarding the use of fat cells in FD.

ARTICLE 116

Ulcerated Lichen Planopilaris of the Scalp: An Hitherto Unreported Clinical Feature and the Successful Treatment by Surgery

Wollina U, Heinig B, Koch A, et al. Ulcerated Lichen Planopilaris of the Scalp: An Hitherto Unreported Clinical Feature and the Successful Treatment by Surgery.
Maced J Med Sci. 2018;6(1):96-8.

Abstract
Lichen planus is a T-cell mediated autoimmune disorder affecting the skin and mucous membranes. Ulcerating lichen planus is uncommon mostly on oral and genital mucosa but not on skin. Lichen planopilaris (LPP), however, is a subtype of lichen planus affecting hair follicles and leading to permanent scarring alopecia. We report a case of LPP of the scalp with multiple alopecic patches ulceration—a hitherto unreported clinical feature. The patient was treated surgically, and the defect could be closed by combined tissue advancement and extension.

COMMENT

Lichen planopilaris (LPP) is a follicular variant of lichen planus characterized by patchy scarring alopecia, erythema and perifollicular scaling. LPP is a follicular variant of lichen planus. It is characterized by lichenoid lymphocytic infiltrates, perifollicular fibrosis, destruction of hair follicles and apoptotic cells in the outer root sheath. Common clinical findings are scarring alopecia, scalp dysesthesia, erythema and perifollicular hyperkeratosis. The disease has a female preponderance and a peak in the fourth to the sixth decade of life. LPP can be subdivided into the following variants: classic LPP, frontal fibrosing alopecia of Kossard (limited to frontal hairline), and Graham-Little syndrome, characterized by multifocal scarring alopecia of the scalp, nonscarring alopecia of the axillae and/or pubis and follicular lichen planus involving the trunk and extremities. While LPP is not known for ulcerations, lichen planus ulcerations may be uncommon but represent a very severe subtype of the disease. This article describes the very unusual presentation, ulcerating LPP of the scalp and the successful surgical treatment.

A 56-year-old postmenopausal female patient with LPP for more than 5 years presented with chronic ulceration of the scalp. On frontoparietal area, a large ulcer measuring 1.5 × 1.5 cm covered with scab was observed. Swab for microbiology revealed large amounts of *Staphylococcus aureus*. After removal of the scab, a scalp ulcer with sharp borders became visible. Complete excision of the ulcer was performed under general anesthesia and lesion was closed after wide undermining of the wound borders by combined tissue advancement and extension using lateral relief cuts. Antibiotic prophylaxis of 1,500 mg cefuroxime was administered 1 hour before surgery. Healing was uneventful and no relapse of ulceration was noted.

Treatment of LPP is usually a medical one with topical or intralesional corticosteroids and topical calcineurin inhibitors for localized lesions. Systemic hydroxychloroquine, methotrexate and cyclosporine A are initiated for widespread disease. Treatment of ulcerative lichen planus needs systemic immunosuppression and often surgery. This case report however does not mention the systemic treatment received by the patient prior or following the surgery.

In long-standing LPP of the scalp, squamous cell carcinoma (SCC) has occasionally been observed. Thus, ulcerative LPP may necessitate histopathological evaluation post resection.

Key Messages

- The lichen planus ulcerations represent a very severe subtype of the disease and SCC to be ruled out in long-standing ulcers
- Treatment of ulcerative lichen planus needs systemic immunosuppression and surgery.

ARTICLE 117

Hair Transplantation for the Treatment of Lichen Planopilaris and Frontal Fibrosing Alopecia: A Report of Two Cases

Liu YS, Jee SH, Chan JL. Hair transplantation for the treatment of lichen planopilaris and frontal fibrosing alopecia: A report of two cases.
Australas J Dermatol. 2018;59(2):e118-22.

Abstract

The current medical line of treatment for lichen planopilaris (LPP) and its variants is limited. Hair growth in the scared tissue is not possible. Hair transplantation restores the hairline and increases hair density but the timing of the transplantation is crucial. Here, we report two Chinese patients with LPP or frontal fibrosing alopecia (FFA) who underwent the follicular unit extraction (FUE) method of hair transplantation after the disease is being stabilized with therapy, with satisfactory results for 3–4 years of follow-up.

COMMENT

Lichen planopilaris (LPP) is subdivided into three variants: classic LPP, frontal fibrosing alopecia (FFA), and Graham-Little syndrome. Medical treatment includes topical or intra-lesional steroids, oral antimalarial agents and tetracyclines that reduce inflammation and stop the disease progression but will not induce hair regrowth from scar tissue. This article reports two cases with LPP and FFA treated with follicular unit extraction (FUE). In the case of LPP, transplantation should only be performed once the disease is stabilized for at least 1-2 years. In this case report, the diagnosis was confirmed by histopathology and FUE was performed after the stability was attained. About 360 and 551 FUs were implanted in FFA and LLP case. During the follow-up, there was no reactivation of the disease and the hair growth was observed after 4-5 months of surgery and both patients followed up to 3-5 years without any complication. Not many studies have documented FUE on patients with LPP. Satisfactory results were obtained with transplantation using the FUE method in the two cases documented in this article.

Key Messages

- Surgical treatment methods for cicatricial alopecia include hair transplantation and scalp reduction
- In the case of LPP, transplantation should only be performed in end-stage alopecic areas and in patients with no disease activity for at least 1–2 years
- The recommended density of the site in the recipient area is 15–30 FU/cm^2 depending on the sufficient blood supply.

ARTICLE 118

Localized Telogen Effluvium Following Hair Transplantation

Loh SH, Lew BL, Sim WY. Localized telogen effluvium following hair transplantation.
Ann Dermatol. 2018;30(2):214-7.

Abstract

Telogen effluvium (TE) is nonscarring type of diffuse hair loss resulting from multiple factors. It is more common in females. The authors have reported two patients who presented with hair loss over the frontal and temporal area after hair transplantation. Histopathology showed normal hair follicle density and increased number of telogen follicles suggesting a diagnosis of TE.

COMMENT

Hair transplantation is a commonly performed aesthetic procedure for androgenetic alopecia. Diffuse hair loss or shock loss is known to occur after transplantation. The authors here have described two cases of localized telogen effluvium (TE) in two patients post hair transplantation. Both patients had noticed acute hair loss 4 and 3 weeks after the procedure and histopathology has shown features of TE.

Possible mechanisms of temporary hair loss following surgery include undue tension at the wound closure site, trauma to follicles, diminished blood supply, stress of operation or emotional stress of being bald prior to surgery.

Awareness of this condition helps the physician to counsel the patient and avoid starting unnecessary medications and surgeries to avoid factors causing TE.

Key Message

- Dermatologists should know and explain to patients that localized telogen effluvium can be the cause of temporary hair loss after hair transplantation and spontaneous recovery of hair loss also happens over time.

INDEX

A

Abametapir 107
Abametapir lotion 106
Abametapir lotion, clinical studies evaluating 105
Abusive attitude 29
Acceptance therapy 28
Acetyl decapeptide-3 99
Achromotrichia 49
Acquired environmental factors 51
Adalimumab 18, 110, 162
Adipose tissue transplant 183, 184
Adipose-derived stem cell 146
Adipose-derived stromal vascular cells 148-150
Albinism 49
Alcohol consumption 49
Allopregnanolone 83
Aloe vera 120
Alopecia 8
  areata 26, 32, 34, 80, 98, 100, 101, 148, 154
    developed 35
    incognita 168, 169
    sparing 35
    tofacitinib for treatment of 95
    treatment of 98, 100
  common clinical presentations 59
  highly effective for 148
  in Association with Malignancy 57
  incidence of 59
  malignancy, treatment-related 59
  multi-centre observational study 59
  neoplastica 58
  risk factors for 59
  survivors of critical illness 59
  tool score, severity of 100
  totalis, case of 80
  types of 60
  use of topical minoxidil in 79
Amino acids 93
Anagen effluvium 57
Anakinra 162
Androgen resistant 181
Androgenetic alopecia 1, 6, 41, 64, 70, 71, 86, 88, 70, 86, 94, 125-128, 135, 136, 154
  drugs for managing 86
  effectiveness for 181
  in male 61, 67, 70
  minoxidil in treatment of 71, 122
  prevalence of 151
  treatment for 61, 68, 122, 146
  treatment of 78, 86
Androgenic alopecia 41
  autologous platelet-rich plasma for treating 129
  technique 8
Antifungal agents 120
Antifungal and anti-inflammatory agents 121
Antihelix 23
Anti-inflammatory agents 120
Antimalarials inhibit tyrosine kinase C 49
Anxiety 88
Apoptotic cells 185
Aspirin 84, 85
Association of Hair Restoration Surgeons 182
Association of Hypothyroidism 43
Atomic force microscopy 4
Atopic diathesis 52
Autoimmune condition, multifactorial 34
Autoimmune disease 32-34, 49
  resulting 32
Autoimmune disorder 158
  chronic 100
Autoimmune T-cell-mediated disease 35
Autoimmunity and nail involvement 32
Autologous adipose derived stem cell 146
Autologous fat transplantation 183
  use of 183
Autologous platelet-rich plasma 129, 133, 145
Azathioprine 100

B

Bacterial
  agent of skin flora 164
  diversity 165
Bar code hair 177
Beck anxiety inventory 119
Beck depression inventory 119
Behavioral avoidance 30
Behavioral based therapeutic techniques 30
Behavioral social avoidance 30
Benign prostatic hyperplasia 82
  treatment of 61
Benzoyl peroxide 120
Bio-based microemulsions 114
Biomimetic peptides 90, 99
Biosimilar adalimumab 110
Biotin 93
Biotinidase 14
Bisabolol cream 121
Black dots 170
Blood
  count 63
  pressure
    diastolic 54
    systolic 54

sugar 51
test 63
Body-focused repetitive behavior disorders 28
Body mass index 51, 116
Body surface area 116
Boggy plaques 23
Burning sensation 184
Burnt matchstick sign 170

C

Cadmium 166
Caffeine-based
  preparation 71
  topical liquid 70
Calcium 49
Calcium pantothenate 50
Cancer therapy 57
Canities 49
Caregivers' sympathy 29
Carpronium 40
Caucasian women 55
Causative fungi 174
Cell proliferation of dermal fibroblasts 91
Cell viability 179
Cellular therapy 148
Cellulitis, dissecting 10
Central nervous system 88
Chemotherapeutic drugs 49
Chemotherapy-induced alopecia 81
Chinese male androgenetic alopecia 141
Chloroquine 49
Cicatricial alopecia 170
Classical lichen planopilaris 43
Clobetasol propionate 114
Cluster of stars 171
Coagulase-negative staphylococci 164
Cobalt 166
Cognitive avoidance 30
Cognitive behavioural
  avoidance scale 30
  therapy 27
Cognitive dysfunction 88
Collagen 93
Colonization of *Pityrosporum ovale* 15

Colonoscopy 18
Color-transition sign 168, 169
Comma hair signs 176
Community dermatology camps, useful in 178
Confocal laser scanning microscopy 73
Confocal microscopy 73
Congenital atrichia with papules 171
Copper 49, 166
Copper peptide 135
Corkscrew hair 170, 174, 177
Crohn's disease 17, 18
Curcumin 111
Cyclic adenosine monophosphate levels 70
Cyclosporine 48
Cyclosporine, treated with 47
Cystic fibrosis 51
Cytopurine 40

D

Deep-dermal mixed inflammation 25
Dehydroepiandrosterone sulfate 63
Demodex mite 164
Depression 88
  anxiety and stress scale 30
Dermal papilla cells 6, 9, 151
Dermatological manifestation of 17
Dermatology life quality index 112
Dermatophyte
  infection, superficial 176
  test medium 23
Dermatophytid reactions 23
Dermo-epidermal junction 173
Dermoscope
  diagnosis easier with 175
  signs 175
Dermoscopy
  for discriminating 174
  forms 178
  in diagnosis 176
Dialectical behavioral therapy 28
Dietary modifications 31

Diferuloylmethane 111
Diffuse alopecia areata 169
Dihydrotestosterone 3, 41, 86
Dihydrotestosterone-induced miniaturization 70
Dilated follicular opening 19
Diphenylcyclopropenone 102
  efficacy of 101
Distal angulation 177
DNA synthesis 80
Donor area 181
Double blinded control trial 134
Dulbecco's modified eagle medium 147
Dutasteride 41, 82

E

Ear sign 23
Ectothrix infection, indicative of 174
Ectothrix parasitation 174
Electrodynamic microneedle 142
  trial of 141
Empathy attitude rather 29
Endocrinal causes 49
Entrapment efficiency 5, 73
Epidermal
  cell 180
  growth factor 89, 128
  melanocyte transfer 180
Epidermis 173, 180
Epiluminescence microscope 173
Epithelial-mesenchymal transition 44
Epithelial stem cells 10
Epithelial-to-mesenchymal transition 10
Erectile dysfunction 88
Erythema 31
Estradiol 160, 161
Etanercept 162
Ethanol 4
Ethosomes 5
Ex vivo drug permeation 73
Excoriation disorder 28, 29
Exogenous oxidative damage 49
Exploratory 29

Extracted follicular outer root
  sheath cell 179
Eyebrow hypotrichosis 81

F

Facial eruptive vellus hair
  cysts 56
Female androgenetic
  alopecia 93
  injections in 132
  platelet-rich plasma on 132
Female pattern hair loss 38, 55,
  63, 66, 72, 77, 125, 155, 156
  combination therapy 65
  controlled study 76
  double-blind 76
  injection on 127
  low-dose oral minoxidil 65
  management of 124
  pilot study investigating 65
  platelet-rich plasma for
    treatment of 126
  treatment course of early 37
Ferritin 51, 168
  low levels of 167, 168
Fibroblast growth factor 135
Fibrosing alopecia 43-48, 55, 80,
  157, 163, 185, 186
Fibrotic scar eventually 23
Finasteride 4, 40, 41, 63, 64, 67,
  68, 76, 86, 136, 154
  administration 42
  adverse effects with 63
  history of 61
  inhibition 89
  loaded ethosomes 3, 4
    evaluation of 3
  long-term side effects of 88
  modified 62
  penetration 136
  risk-benefit ratio of 41
  side effects 42, 63
  solution 87
    use of 87
  treatment impairs
    biosynthesis 88
Fluconazole 22
Fluorescent intensity 5
Folate 167, 168
Folic acid 93

Follicle regeneration 8
Follicle
  stem cell growth 140
  accumulation 155
  keratosis 175, 176
  lichen planus 185
  ostia 55
  plugging 55
  pustules 162, 175
  unit extraction 6, 186
  unit transplantation 182
Folliculitis 19, 23
Folliculitis decalvans 20, 104,
  152, 161, 162, 183, 184
  case of isotretinoin therapy-
    refractory 110
  isotretinoin treatment
    for 104
  recurrent 183
Food and Drug Administration
  6, 141
  adverse event reporting
    system 61
Fractional laser therapy 145
Fractional non-ablative laser-
  assisted drug 135
Fractional technique 136
Frontal fibrosing alopecia 43-45,
  48, 55, 80, 157, 163, 185, 186
Fungal
  culture 25
  epidemic 25
  infections 101

G

Game of time 36
Gamma amino butyric acid
  receptors 88
Gene expression 1, 2, 88
  analysis of 1
Genetic
  hair shaft defects 170, 171
  hypomelanotic disorders 49
Genital defects in the male
  fetus 87
Germinal matrix cells 6, 7
Glutathione 49
Glycemia 63
Glycerin 120
Glycyrrhetinic acid 121

Graham-Little-Piccardi-Lassueur
  syndrome 47
Granulomatous
  dermatitis 23
  infiltrates 23
Granzyme B 34
Griseofulvin 22

H

Habit reversal training 28
Hair
  care products, knowledge
    of 163
  casts 55
  cycling 89
  density, analysis of 155
  dyes 50
  dystrophic 177
  exclamation 170
  follicle 9, 44, 73, 89
    bulge of 10
    growth 151
    immune privilege 34
  stem cells 9, 151, 180
  formulation, intradermal
    injections 139
  growth factor formulation 138
  loss
    cicatricial patterned 55
    female pattern 39, 135
    guidelines for the diagnosis
      39
    male pattern 39, 135
    microneedling for treatment
      of 136
    nanotechnology advances
      for 154
    patches 36
    premenopausal women 63
    treatment of 6, 39
    type of 58
  pull test 128, 177
  pulling disorder 26, 28-30
  restoration surgery 182
  shaft, changes in 170
  transplantation 181, 183, 186,
    187
    controversies in 181
    for treatment of 186
Hairline, designing 182

Harvesting donor hair 182
Head lice infestations 22
   clinical update 21
   treatment of 105
Heavy metal, assessment of 165
Helix 23
Hemoglobin 168
   level 33
Hemorrhagic crusts 162
Herpes zoster 100, 101
Heterozygous male 12
Hidradenitis suppurativa 17, 107-109
Histidinemia 49
Histomorphometric
   evaluation 7
Hodgkin's lymphoma 51
Hoffman disease 17
Homocystinuria 49
Homogenous thickness 177
Hormone levels, range of 160
Human
   autologous adipose-derived 148
   cadaver 5
   follicular phenotypes 6
   hair follicles 1
   hair regrowth, safety and efficacy evaluation 138
   monoclonal IgG1 antibody 117
   oligopeptide-2 139
Hydrophilic drugs 155
Hydroxychloroquine 48, 97
Hydroxychloroquine sulfate 49
Hypomelanotic hair disorders 50

I

Illness, critical 60
Immune
   development 14
   response 15
   adaptive 14
   innate 14
Immunofluorescence
   analysis 7
   microscopy 6
Immunosuppressive like
   cyclosporine 100

Impulse control disorder 26
In vitro drug release 73
Infections, risk of transmission of 132
Infiltrates of neutrophils 23
Inflammasome 161
Inflammasome activation 161
Inflammatory
   cell infiltration 9
   disease, chronic 162
   origin 10
   skin disease 13, 17, 164
Infliximab 18, 162
Inherited seborrheic dermatitis 15
Innate immune signals, activation of 161
Insomnia 88
Insulin-like growth factor 135, 137, 140
Integrin-linked kinase 2
Intensive care units 59
Interleukin, expression of 161
International Society of Hair Restoration Surgery 182
Intracellular signaling pathways 89
Intradermal injections 138
Intralesional injection, effect of 133
Intralesional steroid 48, 183
Intralesional triamcinolone 97
Investigator's global assessment 113
Iron 49, 93, 166
Isomorphic reaction 46
Isopregnanolone regulate specific functions 88
Isopropyl myristate 4
Isotretinoin 47, 105
Itraconazole 22, 25
Ivermectin 22

J

Jakinibs, side effects of 101
Janus kinase 101
Japan Dermatology Association 40
Judgmental therapies 29

K

Keratin 93
Keratinocyte
   growth factor 89, 140
   stem cells 179
   markers of 180
Kerion 22
   surgical drainage of 24
Ketoconazole 24
Koebner phenomenon 35, 46
   case of 45
Koebnerization 47
   phenomena 46

L

Lactoferrin 99, 121
Laser diodes 125
Lead 166
Lesional skin 161
Libido, loss of 88
Lichen planopilaris 10, 11, 44, 45, 48, 97, 157, 162, 163, 186
   activity index 97, 124, 157
   case-control study 43
   characteristics 47
   efficacy of oral tofacitinib 103
   low-level laser therapy in 123
   medical comorbidities in 43
   mild 55
   retrospective study 47
   treatment 47, 103, 186
Lichen planus ulcerations 185
Light therapy, low-level 122
Lindane 21
Linear alopecia areata 36
Lipid
   bilayer 115
   nanosystems 155
Lipophilic nature 155
Lipoprotein
   high-density 51, 54
   low-density 51
Liposome 50
Lithium gluconate 121
Liver
   enzymes 63, 77
   function test 100
   head lice, detection of 22
   human tissue 10

Loose anagen hair syndrome 26, 171
Ludwig pattern 132
Lymphocytes 23
  maintenance of 14
Lymphocytic
  infiltrates 34, 185
  mediated inflammatory, chronic 123

M

Mace hair 170
Maculae cerulea 16
Magnesium 93, 166
Malassezia 120
Malassezia ovalis 121
Malassezia proliferation 120
Malassezia species 164, 165
Malassezia yeast 31
Malathion lotion 21
Male pattern hair loss, topical minoxidil treating 143
Malignancy
  management-related alopecias 58
  status of underlying 59
  type of 57
Manganese 166
Mantoux test 100
Massachusetts General hospital hair pulling scale 30
Mean platelet volume 32
Melanocytes 49, 179
Melatonin 50
Mesenchymal stem cell medium 6
Metabolic syndromes 49
Methionine sulfoxide reductase 49
Methotrexate 47
Metronidazole 121
Microemulsions 115
Microneedling 138
  in alopecia areata 138
  with platelet-rich plasma 129
Microscopic wounds 136
Microsporum 174
Microsporum canis 174, 177
Microsporum infection 174

Minoxidil 1, 40, 57, 61, 65, 70, 73-75, 77, 78, 81, 84
  advantages of 69
  and finasteride, determination of 158
  application 56
  dose of 72
  for androgenetic 68
  in combination 81
  mechanism of action of 1
  method for validation of 159
  oral suspension 74
  percutaneous absorption rate of 142
  side effect of 56
  solution 86, 154
  sulfate, use of 78
  sulfotransferase enzyme 79
  topical solution for the treatment of 141
  uses 72, 81
Mitogen-activated protein kinase 2
Model epithelial stem cell diseases 44
Molecular strata of proteins 50
Monilethrix 81
Monochromatic excimer light 117, 118
Morse-code hair 170
Mud treatment 120
Mutations
  deficiencies in mice 15
  in humans 14
Mycological confirmation 176
Mycophenolate mofetil 47
Myelin protein zero-like 3 15

N

Nanoparticulated systems 155
Nanosystem control drug release 154
Nanosystems promote 155
Narrow-band ultraviolet B therapy 121
National Institutes of Health 71
Neuroactive steroids 88
Neurosteroid
  action of 88
  biosynthesis 88

metabolism of multiple 42
  physiology of 88
Neutrophil count 33
Neutrophilic 23
Niosomes 155
Non-ablative erbium glass fractional laser 135
Nonsocial goals, avoidance of 30
Nonsteroidal anti-inflammatory agents 120
Normal saline 90
Notch and Wnt signaling pathways 2
Novel therapeutic targets 13
Nutritional deficiencies 49, 51
Nutritional supplementation 49, 50, 92

O

Oasthouse disease 49
Obsessive-compulsive
  disorder 119
  spectrum 26
Oil-based nanoparticle 154
Oleic acid 4, 73
  vesicles 73
Oligopeptide 99
Online Mendelian Inheritance in Man 13
Order Derivative Spectrophotometric method 158
Orofacial granulomatosis 20
Oxidative stress 2, 49
Oxidative stress, quantification of 52

P

Panic attacks 88
Pan-Janus kinase inhibitor 97
Paraneoplastic
  alopecia 58
  conditions 57
Park's whorl theory 182
Paternal genome elimination 11, 12
Pathomechanism, underlying 49
Pediculidae 11
Pediculosis pubis 17
Pediculus humanus 11, 12, 21

Pentadecane 40
Perceived stress scale 52
Perifollicular erythema
   and scale 97
   recurrent 162
Perifollicular
   fibrosis 185
   inflammatory infiltrate 23, 162
   vascularization 90, 91
Peripilar sign 170
Peroxisome proliferator-activator receptor gamma 124
Phenylketonuria 49
Pheomelanin production 49
Phosphate buffer saline 4
Phosphodiesterase inhibitor 70
Phospholipids 155
Photodynamic therapy 138, 183
Phototherapy 120
Phototrichogram and trichoscopy 90
Phthirus pubis infestation 16
Phytoestrogens 50
Pigtail hair 170
Pili annulati 171
Pili torti 171
Pilosebaceous unit 3, 4, 7
Piperidino-pyrimidine derivative 75
Plasma cells 23
Plasma rich in growth factors 6, 181
Plasmacytoid dendritic cells 34
Plastic surgery, master of 182
Plastoquinone 50
Platelet lysate 181
Platelet-derived growth factor 128
Platelet-rich fibrin matrix 181
Platelet-rich plasma 98, 126, 127, 131, 145, 146, 181
   effect of autologous activated 127
   injection 146
   meta-analysis on evidence of 131
   plus topical minoxidil 128

Pohl-Pinkus constriction 170
Pollution 49
Polydispersity index 73
Polymerase chain reaction 10, 12
Polymeric nanoparticles 155
Polypeptide growth factors 90
Porfimer sodium 152
Post-Finasteride syndrome 64, 65, 82, 83, 87, 88
   analyses frequency of 64
   clinical manifestation of 87
   drug-induced epigenetics 87
   endocrine disruption 87
   foundation 83
Post-traumatic stress disorder 26
Prader-Willi syndrome 49
Premature aging disorders 49
Progesterone 161
Progesterone level 160
Progressive miniaturization of terminal scalp hair 86
Propecia 62
Propylene glycol 4
Proscar long-term efficacy and safety study 61
Protease production 140
Protein synthesis 125
Protein tyrosine kinases 101
Protein-energy malnutrition 49
Psoriasis 25, 171
   area and severity index 112
   localization of 116
   plaques 35
   scalp severity index 116, 118, 172
Psychological stress environmental factors 51
Pubic and perianal areas 17
Pubis 185
Punishing attitude 29
Pustular dermatosis 58

Q

Quality of life 117
Quantitative telomerase detection kit 150
Quassia amara 120

R

Reactive oxygen species 49
Real-time polymerase chain reaction 23
Red cell distribution 32, 33
Regulatory substances, role of 89
Renbök phenomenon 35
Reproductive system, unusual 11
Retroauricular regions 23
Rheumatoid arthritis 101
Rhodamine red 4
Rough coat 15

S

Sabouraud liquid medium 23
Safe donor area 181
Salicylic acid 85
Salivary sex hormones 160
   correlation of 160
   in trichotillomania 161
Scalp 16, 171, 184
   assessment 140
   biopsy 1, 19, 169, 178
   dermatosis 25
   disorders 171
   dissecting cellulitis of 17
   infestation 171
   psoriasis 117
      desoximetasone topical spray 113
      efficacy and safety 117
      excimer lamp in treatment of 117
      observational study evaluating 113
      open-label 113
      rapid improvement of 116
      retrospective study 117
      treatment 111, 114
   skin 178
Scanning electron microscopy 4
Scarring alopecia 9, 55, 170
   multifocal 185
Seborrheic dermatitis 13, 31, 164, 171, 172
   group 172

lower odds of 31
management of 120
role in development of 165
scalp severity index 172
treatment of 120
Secukinumab 116, 117
Selective Janus kinase inhibitor 1 and 3 100
Selective serotonin reuptake inhibitors 62
Selenium sulfide 24, 121
Self concealment scale 30
Semi-quantitative methods, using of 162
Septic shock 60
Serotonin norepinephrine reuptake inhibitors 62
Serum
 calcium 51
 ferritin 49, 51
 iron 168
Sex hormones, lower levels of 161
Sexual
 dysfunction 88
 hormones 83
 orientation 83
Signaling from stem cells 151
Signaling pathways 1
 activation, examination of 1
Silvery hair syndrome 49
Skin
 disease of 10
 milieu of grafted area 181
 retention 114
Solanum chrysotrichum 120
Solid lipid nanoparticles 154
Soya phosphatidylcholine 4
Spermatocytes, active 12
Spherical morphology 5
Spironolactone 65
Squamous cell carcinoma 18, 185
Stable vitiligo, management of 179
Staphylococcus aureus 20, 164, 165, 183
 infection 152
 role of 152
Starburst pattern 19

Stem cell 8
 based therapies, use of 148
 transition in a human organ 10
Sterile phosphate buffered saline 147
Steroid clobetasol-17-propionate 115
Stimulating hair growth, technique for 123
Stratum corneum 73, 115
Streptococcus agalactiae 20
Stress and anxiety 26
Stromal vascular fraction, adult cells of 148
Suicidal ideation 88
Sulfotransferase enzymatic activity 72
Systemic immunosuppression and surgery 185
Systemic lupus erythematosus 43
Systemic photodynamic therapy 152, 153

T

Tacrolimus 48
Tape stripping technique 73
Tapering hair 170
Targets hair follicles 32
Telogen effluvium 57, 79, 89, 91, 92, 165, 166, 168, 170, 187
 diagnosis of 167
 improvement of 92
 treatment 91
Terbinafine 22, 177
Terminal hair 170
Testosterone 63, 70, 161
 level 160
Thrombocytopenia and neutropenia 101
Thymol 4
Thyroid hormones, decreased 49
Thyroid profile 51
Tinea capitis 18, 22, 18, 26, 170, 174
 children with 175, 176
 clinical recognition of 174
 mimicking dissecting cellulitis 24

monitoring 175
 type of 23
Tissue
 homeostasis 9
 oxygenation 125
Tofacitinib 100, 101
Total antioxidant capacity 31
Trace element levels in patients 165
Traction alopecia 68, 81
Transforming growth factor 89, 128
Trichological disorders, diagnosis of 170
Trichology
 basic 1
 clinical 16
 diagnostic and investigative 154
 surgical 179
 therapeutic 61, 122
Trichophyton
 soudanense 176
 species 25
Trichophyton tonsurans 25, 174
Trichorrhexis nodosa 171
Trichoscope 173
Trichoscopy
 basics of 170
 finding, useful 169
 in pediatric age group 169
 in tinea capitis, utility of 173
Trichotillomania 26, 29, 36
 adolescent females with 160, 161
 assessment and treatment of 28
 clinical characteristics 26
 diagnosis of 160
 ethical considerations 26
 final diagnosis of 119
 incidence of 160
 psychosocial aspects 26
 treatment approaches 26
Trypan blue method 149
Trypan blue staining, using 180
Trypsin-ethylene diamine 179

Tufted hair folliculitis 19
Tulip hair-like structure 170
Tumor necrosis factor
　　inhibitors 18
Turmeric tonic 111

U

Ulcerative lichen planus,
　　treatment of 185
Ultrasound biomicroscopy 125
Ultraviolet
　filters 163
　light, using 152
United States Food and Drug
　　Administration 61
Urea 63

V

Vascular endothelial growth
　　factor 89, 91, 128, 130, 135,
　　137, 139
Vellus hair cyst, eruptive 56
Versus follicular unit extraction
　　182
Vertex and frontal scalp 3
Videodermoscopic analysis 147
Vitamin
　B12 51
　　deficiency of 49
　　levels 167
　D 49
　A 93
V sign 170

W

Wnt signaling pathway
　　activation 151

X

X-linked anhidrotic ectodermal
　　dysplasia 14

Z

Z hair 170
Zero crossing point 159
Zeta potential 73
Zeta potential of
　　polyethersulfone 5
Zigzag hair 177
Zinc 49, 93, 166

EU GSPR Authorised Reprsentative
Logos Europe, 9 rue Nicolas Poussin
1700, La Rochelle, France
Phone: +33 (0) 6 67 93 73 78
E-mail: contact@logoseurope.eu

www.ingramcontent.com/pod-product-compliance
Ingram Content Group UK Ltd.
Pitfield, Milton Keynes, MK11 3LW, UK
UKHW050456150426
5217IPUK00025B/1718